High Intensity Circuit Training

*The New & Advanced Workout
Routine for Burning Body Fat.
Improve Your Fitness Levels, Develop
a Determined Mindset, and Achieve
Your Dream Body in 30 Days!*

By Andrew Hudson

1

acknowledge that the author is not engaging in the rendering of legal, financial, medical or professional advice. The content within this book has been derived from various sources. Please consult a licensed professional before attempting any techniques outlined in this book.

By reading this document, the reader agrees that under no circumstances is the author responsible for any losses, direct or indirect, which are incurred as a result of the use of the information contained within this document, including, but not limited to, — errors, omissions, or inaccuracies.

Table of Contents

Introduction

"I have always got this fat on my belly that seems to never go away. It's always there when I look in the mirror, no matter what I do to try get rid of it, this stops me from having my perfect body and it's so frustrating. The perfect diet is so hard to commit to and I haven't got the time to train for longer. I just want to be able to get my body ready for summer and be proud about it."

This is part of a message that I received from a stranger, that stranger is now a good friend of mine and has been for many years, the reason that the connection was built because I helped her find a passion for living a healthy lifestyle so she could achieve her dream body. As a qualified personal trainer, I have helped many people in this situation and over the years I have been testing and researching the most effective ways for quick yet successful ways to burn fat.

After all the years of research and trying new training methods with my clients and myself, it has been clear to me that HIIT Circuits (A combination of High Intensity Interval Training and Circuit Training) is the most effective training methods to help lower body fat percentage and help people achieve their fitness goals. The best part is, HIIT Circuits can be set up in seconds, completed in under 30 minutes and requires no equipment! I love helping people reach their fitness goal because it lets them experience a range of benefits like an improved mental state, higher energy levels, a better body and much more that you will discover in this book.

You may ask, Andrew if you have found this successful method why are you writing and not coaching people? Well, as I have been stuck at home just like the millions of others, I think there is no better time to write as I can reach a larger number of people in a similar position to you. So that's what I do, I offer fitness help through my books to get people active at home instead of letting them lay on the sofa.

This book is much more than a few exercises written in a list. You will find nutritional information, a guide to the high protein diet, ways to enhance your training, how to go from training once a blue moon to training HIIT Circuits 5 days a week, 5 well-structured HIIT Circuits, motivational advice, meditation and a description for every exercise included in this book. Now that is something I wouldn't miss out on!

It's your turn to take action, however if you turn down this opportunity, although it's hard for me to say this, it is unlikely you will reach your fitness goals and please don't feel the need to live with regret. Instead, you should read this book now and start a new fitness routine as soon as you have finished reading. Exercising gets harder for every day you put it off, so start now! Just give it a real good go, if you can say you've given it a good go, but you didn't enjoy it then fair enough, it's the effort that counts.

Circuit Training for Weight Loss

This is the last book from the three-part series, "Circuit Training for Weight Loss". This series is for people that are looking to reach fitness goals at home with the training method: Circuit Training. Whether your goal is to lose weight to meet job requirements, to improve your health or if you are looking to lower your body fat percentage to look ripped/toned then this series will help you out. Below you will find a brief description of each book and a summary of the series at the end, if you want to find out more, then search up the book titles to view the detailed description!

The first book of these series, it is the most basic, but that doesn't mean that you won't be able to lose weight from it! This book is to get you into a simple exercise routine, will help you clean up your diet and give you an understanding of general health and fitness. This book is a great starting point to set you off on your weight loss journey, helping you break your old unhealthy habits so you can no longer fall under the obese or overweight category.

The second book of the series, "Intermediate Circuit Training", is the next step that increases the difficulty of the workouts, so you make quicker progress towards harder fitness goals. This still sticks with the theme of weight loss with circuit training and nutrition, but this book starts to branch out to slightly more advanced health & fitness information and starts to present motivational advice, so you stay on track with your fitness goal. This isn't for complete beginners, more for the average person looking to lose weight.

The book you are now reading is the final book, "High Intensity Circuit Training", and is the most advanced book. The workouts in these books are shorter, but much more difficult and frequent as this book is to help people with difficult fitness goals like having a low body fat percentage and having a high lean muscle mass percentage. This book also offers advice on how to adapt your mindset to reach challenging goals, information about how to boost your metabolic rate and many other ways to burn fat quickly to lower your body fat percentage while building lean muscle mass. This is for the experienced fitness fanatics.

As you can see, each book from this series is like a steppingstone towards your final fitness goal. Each book goes up in difficulty and if you are looking to go from Fat to Fit, I highly recommend following each book 1 at a time to reach and maintain your goal of having your dream body!

Your Free Gift

The Circuit Training Weight Loss Bundle is a combination of extras to help you reach your goals. These 'extras' can all help in their own way. Below are a few examples of what you may find in the bundle:

- An Equipment Checklist to help you find all the optional equipment that may help you with HIIT Circuits.

- A Calorie Tracking App that makes it very easy to split your diet up and keep on track of what you eat.

- An Extra HIIT Circuit – this one is what I call the Calisthenics HIIT Circuit.

- A Motivational Compilation filled with quotes, something to look at during struggle.

- A HIIT Circuit Cheat Sheet – This makes it easy to refer to the information provided.

You may also find a couple other things hidden in the Circuit Training Weight Loss Bundle…

Follow this link to access the free eBook:

https://hudsonandrew.activehosted.com/f/33

Join the Workout for Weight Loss Community

Living a healthy lifestyle is difficult, especially when you feel as if you are doing it all alone. That's why I suggest for you to join a community of others who are in your situation, this community "Workout for Weight Loss" will provide you with daily posts about weight loss and there will be many people that you can talk to, share experiences with and receive help from.

I aim to post twice a day, providing you with tips, tricks, motivation, workouts, diet plans and so much more to help you lose weight. Not to mention that I may host a few book giveaways every now and then. In a community, your chance of reaching your goals is much stronger and you may make many new friends in the process!

So, if you are looking for that extra help, please join my Free Facebook Group: https://www.facebook.com/groups/workoutfor weightloss

Free "High Intensity Circuit Training" eBook

You may find that in this book there are a few links for you to follow which is inconvenient because you can follow a link through a paperback book without spending 10 minutes typing in 40-character links into your URL.

The links in this book are beneficial to help you progress further with your boxing ability and I don't want you to miss out on them. That is why I am giving you the free PDF eBook copy of this book so that you can access all the links with just a click.

To get the eBook, you will have to type in a short link into your URL (ironic I know...) and you will have the eBook emailed directly to your inbox.

So please type this short link into your internet browser to have easier access to links in this book:

https://hudsonandrew.activehosted.com/f/29

Health Check

Before you start this fitness routine - please consult with your doctor.

- Do not attempt to exercise while unwell.
- Do not carry-on exercising if you feel pain - if the pain doesn't calm please tell your doctor.
- Avoid exercising after consuming alcohol or a large meal within the last couple of hours.
- If you take prescribed medication, check with your doctor to make sure it is okay to exercise.
- If you are in any doubt, go check with a doctor. It may be helpful to show the doctor the circuit training routines you will partake in, if the doctor suggests for you not to partake in certain exercises there are always alternatives that will suit you.

Think before you train. If you are under 16 years old, then I advise you to stay away from lifting weights as your body hasn't fully developed. I 'Andrew Hudson' will not take any responsibility for any physical injuries caused by exercises I have stated in this book – injuries are a part of fitness and can always be avoided so please train responsibly.

Read through the entire book before performing any of the circuits/warmups/cooldowns.

Chapter 1 – What is High Intensity Circuit Training?

Who's This Book For?

High Intensity Circuit Training is a training method that you probably haven't heard of before. HICT is just a mixture of Circuit Training and HIIT, both other these training methods you have probably heard of before. You will probably be able to tell from "High Intensity" that this book provides more advanced workouts for those that are looking to reach more difficult goals. More specifically, this book will help you lower your body fat percentage and gain lean muscle mass so that you look ripped as a man or toned as a woman.

Along your fitness journey you will of course experience many other benefits like improving your fitness level, building mental toughness and much more. So, there is much more than what meets the eye. So, I guess I could say this book is for health & fitness fanatics, although beginners will be able to read and follow this book, I strongly suggest for you to read the last two books of this series if you have less fitness experience.

Whether you want to lower your body fat percentage to look more toned/ripped, or if you want to become fitter because you are training for a certain event, or you just want to lose weight to fit into your favorite jeans. Any reason for wanting to burn fat is a good reason, the HIIT Circuits and advice in this book will help you along that journey. You will find plenty of advanced training advice and information which you can either implement to your HIIT Circuits or other types of training.

This book this the last one out of a three-part book series, the previous two books labelled "Circuit Training for Beginners" and "Intermediate Circuit

Training" both show that this book is the highest level of difficulty when it comes to exercise, meaning this will help those who have more extreme fitness goals and will make a real difference to your training routine. Furthermore, I suggest for those who are less experienced with exercising to check out my previous books of this series before giving this book a real go. That is just a suggestion, if you are a beginner but think HICT is the training type for you then give it a go for it and work towards completing a HIIT Circuit. (A HIIT Circuit is what I call the workouts in this book)

For most of the people reading, I guess you know your stuff when it comes to exercising, of course you can never know everything there is to know in a subject area because new information and research is being carried out each day by the professionals – what I am trying to say here is that I am still able to help you. You are at a level where you will be able to pick up information quickly and use that in your training routine. Even if you are at an average fitness level, you will have more to learn but don't be frightened by that just take it day by day at your own pace.

It is likely that you understand what HIIT is, and you understand how Circuit Training works, don't worry if you are clueless because it's covered in this book. It is likely that you also have a goal you want to reach that involves losing weight, yet again if you don't have a goal, I can help you make one. This book is just more than a Circuit Training guide, it goes much deeper into the mental side of training, provides many tips you can try to reach your fitness goals quicker, contains many facts on why HIIT Circuits are the best way to reach your goals, provides nutritional information and much more.

Circuit Training Basics

Even if you exercise every day without an excuse, it is still possible that you don't know anything about Circuit Training, but I am sure that will soon change. Even if you do know a lot about Circuit Training as you have come from the previous books, I still suggest reading this to solidify your knowledge on the basics.

Circuit training is a workout technique that involves different exercises in a cycle with a rest in between each exercise. Circuits can have between 4 and 12 exercises in a cycle to really give you variety in what you train, there are many variables of the circuit that can be modified to suit you! The variables that make up circuit training and can be changed are:

- **Which Exercises to Include** - This can be any exercise from pushups to burpees, I have included many exercises in this book which require no equipment and can be done anywhere.

- **Number of Exercises in the Circuit** - How many exercises are in the circuit (for HIIT Circuits I suggest 6 to 10).

- **Number of Sets** - Completing a set is where you complete every exercise in the sequence for the required time, this means that if you complete the circuit twice then you've completed 2 sets.

- **Time Spent Doing Each Exercise** - How long you spend carrying out the exercise listed (I suggest around 20 seconds).

- **Time Spent Resting Between Exercises** - This is the valuable time you get for resting between exercises (I suggest 30 seconds).

- **Time Spent Resting Between Sets** - This is the time you have for resting between sets to catch your breath before starting another set (I suggest 1 or 2 minutes).

- **Intensity** - How hard you train (further explained in detail under subchapter intensity).
- **How Many Days a Week you Train** – The number of days a week that you complete a HIIT Circuit.

It is possible to change any variable – this allows for anybody (Beginner or Expert) to be able to complete a circuit as the difficulty of the circuit can be raised or lowered by changing certain variables that I will later explain which variables are the ones that you should change to make the workout more intense, so it becomes a HIIT Circuit. Below you can find a list of benefits associated with Circuit Training:

Circuit Training is Time-Efficient: The circuits in this book are very quick to set up and take around 20-30 minutes to complete.

Circuit Training is Practical: A circuit can be set up anywhere at any time, the circuits in this book require no equipment. Great for Home Workouts!

Circuit Training has Variety: You can fit absolutely any exercise into a circuit so that it allows you to train how you like, for example if you are looking to become stronger you can easily set up a circuit with certain exercises that will work certain muscles. You can also train with the exercises in a different order or train in different areas to provide variety to prevent boredom.

Circuit Training is Easily Modified: If you decide that the circuits provided aren't long enough then you can modify the circuit just by changing how long you spend on each exercise which will make the entire circuit longer.

Circuit Training is for Anyone – Can be done if you are any shape and size because it can be modified to suit you. I take consideration of any difficulties people may face (like joint problems) and I make circuits with exercises that don't require them to bend their joints. This book itself will not contain circuits modified for those with joint problems as they are too intense, refer to previous books. Plus, you will find advice to strengthen joints in this book.

Circuit Training is Fun – This method of training is much different to going on a run. It has a great range of exercises that will get you moving. You can always complete a circuit with another person, you can complete a circuit with music on or anything you like to make it enjoyable for you. If training is enjoyable then you are motivated.

Example Circuit

Here is an example how the circuits are structured and described in this book. I start with listing a few instructions, the first one will be how many sets to complete. Secondly, I state how long to rest in between each exercise – please note that this not the same as the rest period between sets. Think of the rest between sets like Half-time in Soccer, it's a recovery period to prepare you to go again and this usually lasts 1 to 3 minutes. I may also word this as "Rest for 3 minutes after completing the first set". I then set you a target of what heart rate/training zone you should work at. I finally state the time it takes to complete the warmup, circuit and cooldown.

Complete 2 sets, rest for 30 seconds between each exercise with a 2-minute rest between each set. Train at the Light Training Zone

(Around 60% of Max HR). This circuit takes roughly 20 minutes to complete including the warmup and cooldown.

Warmup 4

1. Push-ups – 30 seconds
2. Marching on the spot – 30 seconds
3. Calf Raise – 30 seconds
4. Half Squats – 30 seconds
5. Knees to Chest – 30 seconds
6. Jog on the spot – 30 seconds

Cooldown 3

At the top and bottom of the circuit I include the phrase "Warmup 4" and "Cooldown 3", I have that there because it should remind you to warmup before the circuit and cooldown after the circuit. "Warmup 4" is the name of a warmup I have provided in this book, you will need to be familiar with the warmups and cooldowns I provide in this book as you will be doing them before and after every circuit. If you are confused to where Warmup 1, 2 and 3 are then you would have to look back in the previous books because they suit easier circuits. (Although Warmup 3 is included in this book)

Intensity

Intensity is an important variable that can be changed with ease to modify the difficulty of the training. The first two letters in HIIT stand for High Intensity, that is a big giveaway to how intense your Circuits should be. Before I tell you how hard you should be working, below are the training zones that will be used in this book. As you can see, each training zone is between two percentages of your max heart rate.

Hard Training Zone – 80-90% of max heart rate. You will be breathing heavily and working aerobically. At this intensity you are improving your speed endurance. Lactic Acid will be present in your blood, so training at this zone will allow for your body to handle it well, which will reduce cramps if you consistently train at this intensity. I do not recommend working in his zone for a long period as this may result in injury.

Maximum – 90-100% of max heart rate. Your body will be working at maximum capacity, you can only train in this zone for short periods of time as lactic acid builds up quickly in blood and can cause cramp or injury. The final circuit requires you to work at your Max Heart Rate, so please be careful while in this training zone and make sure to not overdo it.

To go into more detail, the reason why the training zones are determined by percentages of your max heart rate is because it makes the intensity specific to you. To prove my point, if I determined the intensity by asking for 20 jumping jacks in 30 seconds, people who are physically fitter will find that easier because their body has adapted to exercise over time – this means they will be working at a moderate intensity as their muscles don't need as much energy and nutrients that's supplied by blood to complete the 20 jumping jacks. On the other hand, people who aren't as fit will find it harder to complete the jumping jacks in the given time and their heart rate will higher, meaning they are working at a higher intensity.

You will need to be able to measure your max heart rate (HR) to find out what heart rates you should be working between for certain circuits. You can discover what your maximum heart rate is by subtracting your age from 220. For example, if you are 20 years old then you would have a max heart rate of 200bpm (200-20=200).

You will use your max heart rate to work out what heart rate you should be working between. I will use the light training zone as an example here. To find the lower percentage of the training zone (60% for light zone) you will have to divide your max heart rate by 100 and times that new number by 60 (200 / 100 = 2 X 60 = 120 bpm), next you will divide your max heart rate by 100, but times that number by 70 instead of 60 to find the higher percentage of the training zone (200/ 100 = 2 X 70 = 140bpm). If you are 20 years old and looking to work in the light training zone, then you will be lucky enough to have to work in between the nice round numbers of 120bpm and 140bpm.

Why Train HIIT?

HIIT stands for High Intensity Interval Training. This means that the workout will contain short periods of intense and difficult exercise followed by a period of rest or easy and light exercise. Or to put it more professionally – A short work period followed by a slightly longer recovery period. Hopefully, you can already see how this can slide in perfectly with Circuit Training, but before I make the link between the two let's go deeper into HIIT.

HIIT should last no longer that 30 minutes, excluding the warmup and cooldown. This is because your body won't be able to cope with vigorous exercise for too long without risking injury – the recovery period allows you to catch your breath and slightly lower your heart rate to prevent your body overheating, muscles straining or just anything problematic with your body.

Below is a list of the Benefits that come with HIIT:

- HIIT can burn plenty of calories in a short amount of time – this is a massive benefit to those who don't have much time to exercise each day, you can get a brilliant workout in 20 to 30 minutes that will leave you sweating and burning plenty of calories. Researchers found that HIIT burns 20-30% more calories than other forms of exercise.

- Your Metabolic Rate is higher for hours after HIIT – This means that you will still be burning plenty of calories even a couple of hours after you exercise. Metabolism is later explained under the diet section, but I think it's the key for fat burning.

- HIIT can help you burn fat, that may be the most obvious benefit but consistently training HIIT will lower your body fat and the results will come faster than you think.

- You can build muscle with HIIT. That's right, even if you are looking to burn fat training HIIT will allow you to build an amazing physique underneath the layers of fat. The exercises provided in this book may all be body weight, however as you will be completing them at a level of near exhaustion, your muscles will have a harder time exerting and that will make it likely for them to rip and grow back bigger. You should be able to increase your lean muscle mass with HIIT.

- HIIT can improve oxygen consumption, this refers to how well your muscles can use oxygen. It usually takes a very long time of gradual increase of continuous training to increase your oxygen consumption, however it is proven that consistently completing HIIT can provide the same positive results to oxygen consumption in shorter period of time. So, your muscles will be using every bit of oxygen to the best of its ability.

- Can reduce Heart Rate and Blood Pressure – just like most exercise, consistent HIIT training will make you healthier. A lower resting heart rate is great because it shows that your heart is working well and pumping blood around the body efficiently. A lower blood pressure reduces the risk of stroke and kidney disease.

- Blood sugar can be reduced by HIIT and improves insulin resistance. This is very beneficial for those with Diabetes.

Combining the Two

Adding HIIT and Circuit Training together leaves you with HIIT Circuits. These go hand in hand because you can set up your HIIT session in the style of how you can set up a circuit: let me explain further. HIIT Circuits = High Intensity Circuit Training.

If you look back at the sub-chapter "Circuit Training Basics", then you can see that circuit training is very flexible in the way you can train it because of all the variables that you can change. It is very simple to convert a low impact circuit to a high impact circuit by changing the variables – the variables such as intensity will need to be increased and time spent on exercise would need to be decreased. You can of course change other variables if you feel it contributes towards making the HIIT Circuit.

Just to make it clear, a HIIT Circuit requires around 6 to 10 exercises performed at a High Intensity (Above 80% of Max HR) with short periods of rest between exercises and sets. The reason you don't want to have too many exercises in the circuit is because it would most likely put the entire workout longer than 30 minutes and that can be dangerous.

The idea of a HIIT Circuit is to keep your heart pumping quickly for the duration of the Circuit to burn as many calories as you can, which helps you lower your body fat percentage. The HIIT Circuits provided have a large variety of exercises to keep it fun and motivating. A Gym Membership is not needed due to the No-Equipment Exercises meaning that you will save money, plus it saves you from having those embarrassing moments at the gym. Below is a list of benefits which I hope that will urge you to include HIIT Circuits in your training routine, most of these benefits are repeated but it's good to hear it again as it may motivate you more to start using HIIT Circuits.

- HIIT Circuits are time efficient – Under 30 minutes per HIIT Circuit.

- HIIT Circuits are easily set up – Mainly just requires an open space and a stopwatch
- HIIT Circuits are easily modified – There are many exercises and variables that can be changed to make the circuit suit you.
- HIIT Circuits get you into a routine – A key factor to keeping motivated.
- Doesn't have to be done alone – Makes it fun.
- Requires little to no equipment - No equipment is required; however, some equipment is optional as it may provide comfort or help towards your training.
- A real great home workout – If it is cold outside, or the gyms are shut then just find a bit of open space and get started.

HIIT is the most efficient training method to burn body fat. The short periods of intense exercise allow the body to burn calories efficiently without using muscles for energy which allow you to maintain your muscle mass. Longer exercise like continuous training requires more calories to be burned over a longer period and burns away small parts of your muscles to keep your body energized on a long training session. If you want to maintain your muscle mass, then stick to HIIT because the training sessions are shorter and don't rely on muscles for energy.

Extra Information

Here you can find more information that links to HIIT, Circuit Training and so on. Like most things, there is always more than what meets the eye and I hope to have you including HIIT Circuits in your training routine.

HIIT is also a great training method to build lean muscle mass. Although this book isn't focused on bodybuilding or strength training, why wouldn't you want to build lean muscle mass? Firstly, you will be killing two birds by one stone because if you complete HIIT Circuits a few times a week you will be burning fat as well as building/maintaining lean muscle mass – it's such an effective training method. Secondly, the list of benefits of having lean muscle mass is just brilliant. Just look at this list:

- Increased metabolism
- Increased hormonal stability.
- Increased longevity and vitality.
- Reduced risk of illness.

They are just some of the benefits. If you are planning to lose weight and not build any muscle mass, then you will just become skinny. You may think that being skinny is not a bad thing, but it is still unhealthy, unattractive and makes exercise harder to complete as your muscles may be too weak to create movement for a sustainable period.

HIIT Circuits that include explosive bursts of exercise (squat jumps are a good example of these bursts) may be more effective in boosting your V02 Max. V02 Max is the maximum consumption of oxygen measured during exercise, a high V02 Max is very beneficial to your health because it allows more oxygen and nutrients to get to your muscles meaning that your muscles will be able to perform at their best possible ability. Another benefit is that that you will be able to exercise at higher intensities for a longer time before becoming exhausted. Plus, you will be able to hold your breath for longer which can help with meditation and unexpected situations. Your body can use the oxygen more efficiently.

HIIT improves glucose metabolism. Metabolism is explained in the diet section of this book, but to put it simply. An improved glucose metabolism allows for the food you consume (Carbohydrates for this example) to be transferred into energy for your body more efficiently which will help your body and brain function better.

Equipment

Don't worry, <u>not</u> one piece of equipment listed below is <u>needed</u> to complete any of the Circuits. The list of equipment below is all optional, the reason this is included is because each piece of equipment can be helpful towards your training routine.

- Skipping Rope – One of the exercises included in this book can be done with a skipping rope, but it can also be done if you are pretending to skip so it's not needed.

- Fitness Watch – A watch that will accurately measure your heart rate. This can be pricey but will help you manage to train in the correct training zone during exercise.

- Stopwatch – You will just need something to help you keep track of time while training, because it's easy to lose track of time which may mess up the Circuit.

- Fitness Mat – Helpful for when you are completing workouts on the floor, back in the day I used to work out on a towel laid out on the floor!

- Clothing – Just because you are at home doesn't mean you should exercise in your dressing gown. You should have the correct sports clothing when exercising because this will protect you from the environment – for example loose clothing is more likely to get caught on things and heat you up much more than shorts and a t-shirt/top would.

Chapter 2 – The Diet for Effective Fat Burning

As a living being, it is probably a good idea that you eat food. Many people eat because of the feeling of hunger or because they crave a certain food that tastes nice. Although that is a good thing that people eat so that they avoid starvation, eating can become a bad habit because not all food is good for the body.

At the end of the day, food and drink is fuel for the body to keep it working. The body requires a good supply of six essential nutrients to function to the best of its ability. In the previous book "Intermediate Circuit Training" I went into much more detail about these nutrients, what they do, the sources of each nutrient and so on. To keep it short and sweet the six nutrients are:

- Water

- Vitamins

- Minerals

- Fats

- Carbohydrates

- Protein

Energy

I hope that you have heard of each nutrient listed, if you haven't then you will be familiar with the essential nutrients shortly. Each of these nutrients play a large part in providing your body with energy. The nutrients are all found in food, drinks or supplements, so unless you starve yourself then you will be consuming these nutrients on the daily. It is unlikely that you will be severely lacking these nutrients from your current diet, although it is likely that you may not be getting enough of everything which can cause minor symptoms like a lack of energy, dry skin or an itchy scalp.

Your body needs energy for several reasons. The main reason is that your body uses the energy from food and drink to function. The body uses the energy form called ATP (adenosine triphosphate) and this is just like gas in the tank. This gas is used to maintain the body's essential functions like growth, repair, blood transport and it also fuels the muscles and the brain, which is essential to keep you functioning normally, exercising, thinking and so on...

For this book, the main reason for you need to get as much energy in your body as you can because it reflects on how you train. If you can't get enough energy because you don't eat enough, or you eat the wrong kind of foods, or your eating routine is too spaced out then your body will struggle to maintain a good energy level, which will end with you struggling to complete intense exercise.

Energy in food is usually measured by calories. Everyone is different and requires a different number of calories every day, calories are needed for metabolism, physical activity and other things that you may not pay much attention to. The general recommended daily calorie intake for men is 2500 and 2000 for women, as you will want to use every single calorie efficiently to reach your fitness goal then yours will be different. To discover your recommended calorie intake, then you will have to do some maths by following the formulas below:

Adult male: BMR = 10W + 6.25H - 5A + 5

Adult female: BMR = 10W + 6.25H - 5A − 161

W is body weight in kg

H is body height in cm

A is age

I find that a weird formula, but most importantly it allows for you to work out your Basal Metabolic Rate, you will learn more about this under the subchapter metabolism however for now you will need you BMR to insert into the formulas below. Please only select one of the options that applies to your current exercise situation.

1. If you are moderately active (moderate exercise/sports 3-5 days/week): Calorie-Calculation = BMR x 1.55

2. If you are very active (hard exercise/sports 6-7 days a week): Calorie-Calculation = BMR x 1.725

3. If you are extra active (very hard exercise/sports & physical job or 2x training): Calorie-Calculation = BMR x 1.9

Now you will have a number which is specific to you, this is the number of calories that you should aim to consume every day. This is the energy your body needs for functioning, for exercise and other things. You don't have to make sure you consume that exact number of calories each day, as long as it is close enough then it will help you burn fat, build lean muscle and provide your body with energy. If you exercise less than 3 times a week then that's what you should work towards before getting into HIIT Circuits!

High Protein Diet

I would like to firstly clear something up, when I say you should try get as much energy as you can into your body – I do not want you to constantly stuff your face with snacks and treats, just because they may be high in carbs and provide plenty of energy doesn't mean it will be good for you.

Instead, you have to split up your diet. The reason why you want to split up where you get your energy from is because that not all energy sources are good for the body, some nutrients that provide energy may be good for you but once you have too much then that excess energy will be stored as excess fat.

As you are soon to be HIIT Circuit experts, I suggest you follow a high protein diet plan. The High Protein should be made up of around 40% of foods high in protein, 30% of foods high in fat and 30% of foods high in carbohydrates. Use calories as a system of measurement, I previously asked you to work out your recommended calorie intake and now you will have to split it up to meet these requirements. I say around 40% for foods high in protein because that should allow you to reach your recommended protein intake for if you are building muscle. Even if you do not want to build muscle - I still suggest a high protein intake because it plays an important role in your body and excess protein isn't harmful. Below you will find all the previous six essential nutrients which are all explained briefly on how they work and where they can be found (more information in previous books).

40% Protein – Foods that are high in protein basically make up this diet plan, so that's why just under half of your day will consist of eating foods high in protein. This may seem like too much protein, and for those of you who have low muscle mass then it is too much. Fortunately, too much protein doesn't do any harm apart from making your farts stink – yep that's true. So, make sure you have at least 40% of your daily diet covered by protein but the more you have is better and will keep your muscles strong.

Your body needs around 1.2g – 1.7g of protein per kilo of your body weight so that the muscles can grow and repair stronger after exercise, using myself as an example 80kg x 1.5 = 120 grams of protein every day. Unfortunately, consuming all this protein will not automatically make you look like Arnold Schwarzenegger – you will have to complete exercises consistently which cause the muscle to rip slightly so it can grow back stronger. Although I don't think you should worry about building muscle too much, if you stick to this diet and a training routine with HIIT Circuits I am sure you will have no trouble gaining lean muscle mass – if you are worried about gaining too much muscle mass the body weight exercises won't allow you to build too much!

Foods that are high in protein can be found here: Eggs, lean meats, poultry, salmon, beans, cheese, and natural peanut butter. With there being many more foods out there with similar protein properties. I also find protein shakes to be incredible protein providers. High protein foods are filling and make it harder for you to snack due to your filled stomach.

30% Fats – A decent chunk of the high protein diet should come from fat, this may sound stupid if this book is all about burning fat but let explain why this is the case. Firstly, you will find that some of the foods you consume that are high in protein are also reasonably high in fat – foods high in protein and fat will fill you up, will provide your body with enough energy and make it less likely for you to snack throughout the day.

There are good fats and bad fats, you will want to include both types into your diet but ideally consume more good fats than bad fats. The good fats are called: Polyunsaturated fats and Monounsaturated fats. While the bad fats are called: Saturated fats and Trans fats. You need to break up roughly how much of each you consume.

Out of the 30% for you daily fat intake, I would suggest for you to have 20% of that from the good fats and 10% from the bad fats.

Monounsaturated fats (good fats) are found in nuts, vegetable oils, peanut butter and avocados. While Polyunsaturated fats (good fats) are found in oily fish: Salmon, Herring, Trout, Sardines, and tuna, as well as tofu, walnuts, flaxseeds, vegetable oils and seeds. These good fats should make up roughly 20% of your daily diet, these will help reduce heart discase, lower the bad cholesterol and provide many health benefits.

Trans fats (bad fats) are found in fried food (doughnuts, fast-food), margarine, baked goods (cakes, pastries) and processed snack foods. You need to avoid Trans Fats because they provide no nutritional value and are damaging to the body – save these foods for the cheat day! Saturated Fats (bad fats) are found in high fat meats and dairy products such as: beef, pork, dark poultry, lamb lard, cheese, whole milk and tropical oils. 10% of your daily diet should come from Saturated Fats because your body needs fat for energy, and you will find it very hard to eat all that protein without consuming any saturated fat.

30% Carbohydrates – This diet plan requires a lower amount of carbohydrates than usually recommended, this may be a difference to your current diet because carbs usually make up a large part of our daily diet. Carbohydrates can be split into three types: sugar, starch and fiber. These carb types are either 'Simple carbs' or 'Complex carbs' because of how your body can deal with them for energy.

Simple carbs are easy to digest and are a good source of energy – natural simple carbs may be simple sugars found in fruit and added simple carbs are found in processed food or refined sugars like cake or sweets. Simple carbs are a good source of energy, but you have to stay away from the 'added sugars' because these are more likely to cause your blood sugar levels to spike which increases your appetite – "added sugar" carbohydrates are known as empty carbs because of they offer little nutritional value apart from a good taste. If you consume lots of foods high in protein then you will have an easy time cutting down the amount of simple carbs you have, I think Fruit and Lucozade are great sources of simple carbs that will help you get the energy you need.

Complex Carbohydrates take longer to be digested because they are formed in long complex chains. Complex carbs can be found in foods like wholemeal bread, wholemeal pasta, barley, quinoa, potatoes and corn. Complex carbs are rich in nutrients because they contain vitamins, minerals and fibre. Fiber is a brilliant nutrient because it fills you up, from the 30% of carbs that you will consume on the daily make sure to check the packing and look out for the foods highest in fiber because that sure will stop you snacking.

All carbohydrates are converted into glucose within the body, which is blood sugar, however depending on how easy they are to digest depends on how long it takes for the sugar to get into the blood. The simple carbs almost convert to glucose immediately, consuming a large amount of simple carbs is likely to increase your body fat percentage as the excess glucose that is not used by the body is converted to glycogen and is later stored as fat. Complex carbs provide your body with energy for a longer time period because of how long the take to digest, this is better for your body because it will keep you energised for longer and reduces snacking.

Complex carbs are a better source of energy for your body, but simple carbs from natural sources are also a good quick energy boost before a workout if needed. So, I suggest for you to have 5% of your daily calorie intake come from simple carbs such as fruit, milk or Lucozade's because these are the better options for simple carbs which contribute towards high energy levels. Please avoid the added sugars like cakes because they don't provide any sustainable energy. The other 25% should come from Complex Carbs, these will allow for you to maintain high energy levels throughout the day and reduce your appetite to reduce snacking.

Vitamins – Vitamins play a large part in the body as they perform hundreds of roles like bolstering your immune system and healing wounds. It is important you get a good supply of all the essential Vitamins like Vitamin A, Vitamin D, Vitamin K and so on. If you are sticking to this high protein diet, exercise regularly and go outside regularly then you won't fall short and should avoid the symptoms like having a lack of energy, or having poor vison. To be certain that you get all the essential vitamins you need to function to the best of your ability then I suggest taking Vitamin and Mineral tablets.

Minerals – Minerals are important because they keep your body functioning properly. Just like with vitamins, there is not really any reason to worry about consuming minerals as it is likely to be found in your food and drink. To ensure that you get all the minerals that you need (there are quite a few) then I would suggest taking vitamin and mineral tablets every morning.

Water – It is very important to stay hydrated. A good way to indicate whether you are hydrated is by looking at your pee, if your pee is transparent then you are hydrated, and your body would have flushed out the toxins and the water in your body can help transport nutrients around the body efficiently. However, if your pee is yellowish then that is a sign you are dehydrated and need to consume more water. Enough about pee, here are the facts you need. You should consume over 3 litres of water every day. Get into a routine of drinking water consistently throughout the day, don't try to drink 3 litres at once because that is extreme. Always have a glass/ bottle of water present when exercising because that is when your body needs water the most.

Calorie Intake

This is an example of my calorie intake and how I would split it up every day between fats, carbs and protein. I am 180cm in height, 26 years old and 80kg in weight. So that means to work out my recommended calories I would do the following:

(10x80kg) + (6.25x180) − (5x26 years old) + 5 = 1800BMR.

I would then take that number then times it by 1.725 (I am very active, exercise 6-7 days a week) which means I would have to consume 3105 calories every day. That may be a lot, however I am very active with a muscle mass percentage higher than the average person, so keep that in mind.

Here is a website that you can use to measure your Calorie Intake which is much simpler than following that formula previously mentioned: https://www.calculator.net/calorie-calculator.html.

On this website you should be able to put in your info and click calculate to find your recommended calories intake, this will give you the same number as working out the formula. After that you will see a table with 4 different numbers on there, the highest number is your recommended calories which means if you consume that much following the high protein diet, they will maintain your body weight (you will burn fat but

64

build lean muscle mass as a weight replacement which is great).

Below your recommended calories you will see another 3 numbers which are lower than your recommended intake, for me those numbers are 2856 calories, 2606 calories and 2105 calories. By reading the chart you can see these are the calories you would have to consume to lose weight at a particular rate. I do not recommend following the bottom figure because there should be no need for you to lose weight at an extreme rate.

I suggest you either pick to eat your recommended calories for maintaining weight or to eat your recommended calories for mild weight loss. To continue using myself as an example, I will follow my recommended intake for mild intake which requires me to follow this formula:

(Recommended Calorie Intake for Maintaining Weight) x 0.92 = Recommended Mild Weight Loss Calorie Intake.

3105 Calories x 0.92 = 2856 Calories

Eating this number of calories will allow me to burn fat and lose a small amount of weight each week. At some point though you will have to eat the recommended amount to maintain weight because losing too much weight may not be what you are after. Below you can see how I can split up my day of eating to reach the 2856 calories.

40% of my daily diet will be made up of foods high in protein which means that I would consume roughly 1150 calories worth of lean meat, eggs, protein shakes, milk, beans, fish, cheese and other foods high in protein throughout the day. I make sure to have a large variety of proteins to make my day of eating enjoyable. Most importantly, I would make sure I meet my recommended protein intake for building muscle.

30% of my daily diet will consist of foods high in fat. More importantly 20% of the Good fats and 10% of saturated fat which would equivalate to around 300 calories of saturated fat and 600 calories from the Good Fats.

30% of calories come from Carbohydrates. To be more specific 5% will come from Simple carbs and 25% will come from Complex carbs. So roughly 100 calories worth of Simple but natural carbs and around 650 of calories from Complex carbs.

That is everything split up, it is now your turn to find out how many calories you require and how you are going to split it up. This is also a good place to address a cheat day, a cheat day is a day where you can enjoy all the foods you have been trying to resist because of how unhealthy they are. A cheat day once a week/two weeks is great because it gives you something to look forward to.

I don't need you to be exact with the calories you consume, as long you are within 50 calories for each requirement then your body will begin to make the positive changes. My day adds up to around 2800 calories which is good enough because remember you are still doing the exercise to help you get towards your goal.

High Protein Diet Benefits

Below is a list of benefits of the High Protein Diet. I hope for this to prove why a high protein diet is the best option for those who want to burn fat quickly.

- Protein rich foods will reduce your appetite which will naturally prevent you from snacking and cravings. (Regular snacking is linked to putting on fat quickly)

- Protein is the building block of your muscles. A high amount of protein in your diet will allow you to build up lean muscle mass and become stronger as the circuits provide exercises that exert your muscles.
- Good for your bones as protein helps increase calcium absorption.
- Protein boosts metabolic rate by 20-35%, this will help your body burn calories more efficiently.
- Lowers blood pressure – a real good benefit to your overall health.

There are many other diet plans out there to help with fat burning, which I believe for the keto diet to be very popular at the moment. If you don't think the high protein diet will benefit you then feel free to follow a different diet plan that suits you. I understand some of you reading may be vegetarians or lactose intolerant which does restrict where you can get your protein from – although it doesn't make it impossible, so do your best to get all the protein you need.

Foods to Avoid

Straight to the point, below are foods and drinks that you should cut out from your diet. If you really struggle to resist the urge to eat these treats, then I am sure a cheat day once a blue moon won't hurt. Life is too short to constantly restrict yourself of these treats – as long as you make sure it is only once a blue moon.

- Foods and drinks high in sugar – like Coca Cola, Chocolate, Sweets, Cookies are all high in sugar. These treats will cause spikes in your blood sugar levels that cause hunger and as we know hungry people just keep eating and keep gaining weight. The excess glucose from the sugary foods is stored as glycogen in the liver – overtime this turns into fat which will make your belly look rounder.

- Alcoholic drinks – Wine, Beer, Spirits are all bad for you. Now if you enjoy a drink or two like me, then cut down on how often you have a drink and arrange for a night to drink once a blue moon (maybe on your cheat day?). Drinks that contain alcohol are not good for you because alcohol contains many toxins that are damaging to the liver, the heart and the effects of alcohol can damage your mental health over the long term. So, enjoy a glass every now and then, just don't drink consistently.

- Processed food (if you can) – Unfortunately, it is very difficult to go a day without eating something that is processed. Processed foods contain high amounts of added sugar, fat and sodium which isn't want our body wants in large quantities. Plus, I couldn't even begin to tell you all the ingredients they use for some processed foods, some of the stuff sounds like elements off the periodic table!

- Snacking – I understand that there is no food out there called "Snacking", but this is included because it is vital that you cut down on all the treats and snacks throughout the day. It is common to get the urge to enjoy a quick chocolate bar or cookie because it tastes nice and when you are bored eating helps pass the time. One snack a day which is healthy will do no harm - examples of healthy snacks include nuts, a handful of berries, natural Greek yogurt, or Apple slices with peanut butter.

- Fruit Juices – This often catches people out because fruit is healthy right? Well yes, but not fruit juice. Most fruit juices have lots of added sugar and one glass of apple juice can contain enough sugar that you need for a day. So, limit how often you have fruit juice or just drink fruit juice without added sugars.

Good foods for your Brain

Your brain is what controls your thoughts, memory, speech, movement, the function of your organs and much more. So, it is important we get the brain what it needs right?

Oily Fish – Be sure to include oily fish into your diet as they include a high amount of fat, protein and omega 3. The unsaturated fats found in the fish lower the blood levels of beta-amyloid (this is a protein that forms in the brain and is damaging). Eating oily fish a few times a week can improve brain power and reduce the risk of Alzheimer's disease. Examples of oily fish: salmon, cod, tuna and pollack.

Green Leafy Vegetables – These vegetables are high in Vitamin K, lutein, folate and beta carotene which are all brain healthy nutrients. Examples of leafy green vegetables are kale, spinach, collards and broccoli – I would suggest including these on the side of a high protein meal because I can't imagine Kale being enjoyable on its own.

Berries – Berries are great for you but in low quantities because they are simple (although natural) carbs which will spike your blood sugar level. Let me get to the reason why they are great, simply because they are loaded with antioxidants. Antioxidants help protect the brain cells from damage which will keep your thinking sharp and knowledge maintained.

Tea + Coffee – Tea has caffeine and L-theanine while coffee contains caffeine. These drugs (legal drugs) are good for the brain because they promote central nervous system stimulation. This means that alertness and focus of the brain is increased over a short period of time. This is the important part, please limit your intake of caffeine because too much is dangerous. Having a cup of coffee late at night will keep you awake for a long while, which may mess up your sleeping pattern. I am sure that some of you enjoy a cup of coffee as soon as you wake up, which is great, stick to a cup a day and look out for the training tips section in the next paragraph to learn how caffeine can help you with exercise and fat burning.

Remember to take these into consideration with your diet plan, don't go constantly stuffing your face with oily fish because your body will lack the nutrients that the oily fish don't provide, it's all about splitting up your day of eating to meet the nutritional requirements. If your brain is healthy, then you will be healthy.

Metabolism

Your metabolism is a term to describe all chemical reactions involved in maintaining the living state of the cells and organisms. The three main purposes of the metabolism are to: convert food to energy to run cellular processes, convert food to building blocks, and finally the metabolism has the purpose to eliminate metabolic waste. Overall, your metabolism is what converts food into energy.

Everybody has a different metabolic rate, the metabolic rate is the speed that the metabolism works at. Those of you who have a quick metabolic rate will be able to eat a lot without gaining weight because your body can burn more calories easily, while unfortunately those with a slow metabolic rate will find it easier to put on fat as not all the calories burn easily and the left-over calories store as fat. If you know you have a slow metabolic rate or you don't know your metabolic rate, it is still possible for you to burn fat, you will have to increase your metabolic rate. Before I get into that, you should know the categories of metabolism.

Basal Metabolic Rate (BMR) – This is your metabolic rate during sleep or deep rest. Your body is always working even at rest to make sure everything is functioning well, and this is the minimum calories needed to keep your lungs breathing, to control body temperature, to keep the heart beating and the brain fully functioning. Remember this is used to measure your daily calorie intake.

Resting Metabolic Rate (RMR): This is the lowest possible metabolic rate to keep your body functioning. This accounts for 50-75% of total calories used.

Thermic Effect on Food (TEF): This is the number of calories burned while your body digests food. This usually takes up around 10% of total calories used.

Thermic Effect of Exercise (TEE): Calories burned while exercising. This is something that will be high for all of you if you exercise HIIT regularly.

Non-Exercise Activity Thermogenesis (NEAT): This is the number calories required for simple activities such as standing, walking, fidgeting etc.

All the above contribute to how all the energy (calories) that you consume is being used every day. There are many contributing factors that affect your metabolic rate. A list of these is below, some of them are unable to be changed however I later suggest how you can make a change to these contributing factors to speed up your overall metabolic rate.

- Age – The older you are the lower your metabolic rate is. You are unable to go back in time unfortunately, however, don't let this put you off making an effort to increase metabolic rate, just see this as an obstacle if you are in that position.

- Muscle mass – The more muscular you are, the more calories you burn because your bigger muscles need more energy to maintain size and be used.

- Hormone disorders – Cushing's Syndrome and Hypothyroidism slow down your metabolic rate. For those that suffer with these disorders, don't let it stop you from training and increasing metabolic rate.

- Physical Activity – The more active you are, the more calories you burn. This factor can link to muscle mass as exercise allows for muscle mass to be increased.

- Temperature – When you are exposed to cold temperatures then your body needs to work harder and burn more calories to stay warm. But please don't feel the need to move to the artic, maybe just a cold shower everyday may help with this.

To help you lower your body fat percentage, lose weight or whatever your fitness goal is I suggest for you to try to increase your metabolic rate. This will allow you to burn more calories which will burn fat, will allow for you to maintain high levels of energy and below you can find a list of ways to increase metabolic rate which also contain their very own benefit to you mentally or physically.

- Consistent HIIT exercises – I mean this book alone covers all the benefits of HIIT Circuits and you will be able to try the HIIT Circuits included in this book to really see if they bring the positives mentioned.

- Consistent eating – By this I mean that you should space out your day of eating into 5 smaller meals to avoid going into starvation mode. Starvation mode is what your body goes into when you haven't eaten in a while and your body has to adapt to the lack of energy, which decreases your metabolic rate and also makes your body burn your muscles for energy, which lowers your muscle mass. So, avoid this starvation mode and eat regularly throughout the day to maintain a high metabolic rate. Don't stick to 3 meals a day!

- Eat lots of protein – This will be easy for you if you follow the high protein diet.

- Drink more water – Drinking water over sugary drinks is good for you because drinking at least 3 liters of water a day can increase metabolism by 10-30%.

- Drink Green Tea or Oolong Tea – These teas help convert some of your fat stored in your body into fatty free acid which increases fat burning by 10-17%.

- Eat Spicy Foods – Although I cannot take the heat, peppers contain capsaicin which can boost your metabolism. If you cannot handle the spice, then I understand if you avoid this because I can't handle it either.

All the methods above to increase your metabolic rate work differently for individuals, but if you want to get the best results you can then I suggest sticking to as many as them as you can – plus you will find yourself doing some of them naturally when in a fitness routine.

When's the Right Time to Eat?

To be honest, there is not an exact answer to this question, but it is important you structure out your day of eating. Eating 5 or 6 smaller meals throughout the day is proven to provide many more benefits to your health and helps boost your metabolism compared to eating 3 meals a day. Try to leave around 3 hours between each meal, I will give an example of how to space out each meal:

1. Breakfast – Between 6am and 9am.

2. Mid-morning Meal – Between 9am and 12pm.

3. Lunch – Between 12pm and 3pm.

4. Mid-afternoon Meal – Between 3pm and 6pm.

5. Dinner – Between 6pm and 9pm.

Look at that! A great way to balance your day of eating out. If you like a healthy snack or two then feel free to snack between meals (if you are not training at that point) or before bed – just take into consideration the size of your snack.

Eating around a HIIT Circuit needs consideration. Eating too soon before or after a HIIT Circuit will most likely end with you vomiting because your body would not be able to digest food properly due to your high heart rate. I suggest that you consume a meal roughly 60 to 90 minutes before a HIIT Circuit, or you can consume a light snack around 30 minutes before if it fits into your eating routine. A pre workout meal or snack needs to be able to provide your body with enough energy to go ahead and complete the HIIT circuits. I feel slightly guilty for not providing many food examples in this book, so below is a list of light but healthy snacks/meals to enjoy roughly 30-90 minutes before a HIIT Circuit:

- Sliced banana on a rice cake.
- Greek yogurt with berries.
- Whole grain toast with nut butter or sliced meat.
- Oats with dried fruit.
- Hummus and pita bread.

It is a good idea to have a snack/meal after a HIIT circuit to replenish your body with nutrients and energy, this will also help with recovery. Here are a few meal ideas for 30 minutes after a HIIT session:

- Egg white omelet loaded with vegetables and a side of fruit.
- Peanut butter and banana in a whole grain wrap
- Oats with a banana and yogurt.
- A chicken or turkey sandwich wrap.
- Protein Shake with strawberries.
- Lean meats with quinoa and vegetables.
- Whole grain toast with peanut butter.

Chapter 3 – How to Enhance Your Training

As you will be training at the top level, this chapter is dedicated to helping you exercise to the best of your ability to speed up progression towards your goal. You will find training tips to help you when it comes to exercise, goal setting techniques to refuel your ambition and plenty of other tips to contribute towards your goals.

Rest and Recovery

Resting and recovering is needed after a workout, especially when it comes to High-Intensity-Interval-Training. Whether you are training HIIT 4 days a week or 7 days a week then it is important you do the best you can to rest, recover and prepare for your next circuit. That's the main reason you want to rest and recover because if you have got a HIIT Circuit to complete in 30 minutes, but you are still knackered and aching from the HIIT Circuit you completed yesterday, then you will struggle to keep the training up to standards. Not to mention that rest and recovery prevents injury.

Below you can find a few ways which help your body recover after training, I expect you to follow most of these tips because if you don't then you simply won't be able to reach your goal.

- Rest – It's in the title. After a circuit, it's good to relax to lower your heart rate and take the stress of your muscles. Sleep is a big part of rest; you need 8 hours of sleep every night so that you can wake up feeling fresh and energized for the next day of exercise.

- Cooldown – A cooldown needs to be performed straight after the circuit. The benefits of cooldowns are explained in chapter 5. Just get into the habit of cooling down after exercise, if you don't then your body will have a hard time adapting to the sudden change in heart rate.

- Stay Hydrated – While you are exercising you should always have a bottle of water laying around because you will be sweating, and the lost water needs to be restored. Also have a glass of water after a workout because you may still be sweating for a short while afterwards and you need to replace the lost fluid.

- Eat your proteins – As you are likely to be following a high protein diet then this will be easy for you. Getting in protein will help rebuild your muscles that have been slightly damaged during the workout.

- Electrolytes – As you sweat you lose electrolytes which are things like potassium, sodium chloride, magnesium and calcium. A light snack like fruit or a sports drink like Lucozade after the workout will replenish your electrolytes. It is common for electrolyte loss to cause cramps which you will want to avoid.

- Have a Proper Rest Day – May be difficult for those who exercise 7 days a week, but eventually you will have to give your body one full day to relax. A gradual buildup of stress and tension from exercise over a long period of time can set you up for a long-term injury in the future. If you do plan to exercise 7 days a week, try to fit in a rest day once a fortnight. In other words, don't let your mindset make you overtrain.

- Get a Massage/Myofascial Release – These methods are ways to physically take stress away from any sore muscles. A massage improves circulation which allows you to relax and it helps the muscle recover. Myofascial release is like giving yourself a massage with a foam roller, you roll the foam roller over the muscles that ache, and it will help improve circulation within that muscle.

- Ice Bath – A very popular recovery technique. Getting in and out of an ice bath will cause a sudden change in temperature meaning that our blood vessels constrict and dilate repeatedly. This is meant to flush out waste products in tissues causing a quicker recovery.

The tips above will help you increase your recovery time and prevent injury. The quicker your recovery time then the less time it takes for your body to repair from the previous workout. Once you have a great recovery time you will be able to exercise HIIT every day without a problem, if you are looking to train twice a day using HIIT Circuits and Weight Training then feel free but you must consider the muscle groups you are using, don't go all out by completing exercise that only use your arm muscles because the excess tension on your arm muscles may cause injury.

Progressive Overload

Progressive overload is a key factor to use when it comes to making gains – whether that is to gain muscle mass, improve endurance or burn fat. I have used progressive overload in all my circuit training books with the six-week plans to help you make progress. Unfortunately, you will not be able to find a six-week plan in this book as I believe you can use the structure from the last two books to make your own specific training plan.

Enough of six-week plans. Progressive overload is where you increase the workload of the circuit overtime by increasing or decreasing variables. I like to use the Jumping Jack example to explain progressive overload. If you have an overweight person and an athlete in the same room and told them to complete 20 jumping jacks in 30 seconds then the overweight person will struggle to complete it and the athlete will be able to do it easily, right?

As the overweight person may not be used to exercise and weighs more, that means their heart must pump faster to pump more blood around the body to the muscles due to the workload, meaning that he has a higher heart rate. As the athlete's body has adapted to exercise then their heart rate would be lower, this means they must increase their workload to match the overweight persons heart rate.

This means as you get fitter from exercising and eating well then you will have to increase your workload over time so that you can maintain your heart rate for every HIIT Circuit session, the ways to increase the workload of a HIIT Circuit include:

Increasing time spent for each exercise – Only increase this variable by a second or two at a time because working at a high intensity for too long is risky. But increasing this by a couple seconds will maintain your high heart rate for longer which ends up with more fat burned.

Decreasing your rest period – Yet again, only decrease this for seconds at a time because resting between High Intensity Exercises is vital for recovery. Having a shorter rest period will give your heart rate less time to slow down meaning the workload is increased.

Increasing Heart Rate – Quite obvious, but if you manage to exercise at a faster pace, that will cause your heart to beat faster meaning you are increasing the overall workload of the HIIT Circuit.

Using Equipment – This doesn't apply to the exercises in this book, but it is a great thing to know because if you start using weights for some of the exercises, then the resistance caused by the extra weight will force your muscle to work harder, which means your heart pumps faster.

It is up to you to know when to use progressive overload in your training routine. Making a small change every week to your circuits that increase the overall workload, will help you reach your goals. Without progressive overload you may find yourself at a stage where you are not burning fat as effectively as you were at the beginning, once you reach your goal and want to maintain that goal then progressive overload is not as important. But I suggest you slowly increase the overall workload of your HIIT Circuits over time, remember that the circuits I have included are all at different difficulties so keep that in mind.

Injury

Injury is a setback. I am sure many of you that have been training for years have been injured in the past and you know how unfortunate it is. While training at a top level, it is more likely for you to get injured due to the intensity you will be training at, that's why it is vital I cover the best tips to avoid injury.

- Warmup before Circuits. This is hopefully screwed into your brain by now.
- Cooldown after Circuits – Again will be screwed into your brain.

- Don't train if you feel a slight pain – Training with a slight injury makes it worse.

- Don't work too hard for too long - Very important in this book. I advise you not to massively increase the length of time that you are exercising for as your body will find in hard to cope.

- Wear appropriate Clothing/footwear – Wearing normal clothing may cause you injury because the grip on your footwear may cause you to slip or your top may be too baggie and get caught on an object.

- Stay hydrated/eat correct foods.

- Allow time to recover after training.

- Develop the correct mindset – Chapter 8 is heavy on mindset for a good reason. Because those of you reading this may be excited to train HIIT and may go "Over the Top", by this I mean people are so motivated to reach their goal that they put in extra training on rest days and push their body to the complete max. Although I like the motivation, you should know training too often links to injury – much more is said in Chapter 8 and hopefully will help you find your balance of training.

- Complete Proper Form – I hope that after reading Chapter 7, you will have no issue with form. However, it's a good idea to practice exercises until you get it right before using them in a HIIT Circuit, because if you complete an exercise at a high intensity with the incorrect form that is likely to make you use your muscles out of balance – extra exercise on muscle groups because of balance issues may cause injury.

In Chapter 8 you can find plenty of information about an injury setback plan which is under the subchapter "More Motivation". To put it shortly a setback plan is a plan for how you will cope under the unfortunate circumstance of injury, this plan will help you turn a bad situation into a learning process and come back stronger than ever before.

In my previous books I have always covered how to prevent injury and it is hard for me to come up with new ideas to do with prevention as there is only so much you can do, but here you can find ways to deal with injuries. Whether the extent of your injury is small or large I am sure this may help. As injuries aren't always possible to avoid, below is a list of ways to treat injuries:

- Stick Ice on it – Cover an icepack with a towel and rest it on the part of your body which is injured. Applying a cold object to the injury will reduce inflammation and numb the pain.

- Rest – Every day should be a rest day unless you can exercise without using the injured part of your body (check with doctor).
- Ibuprofen – This is a painkiller that will reduce the pain and bring down swelling. Yet again I advise you to check with your doctor because I don't know your medical history and certainly don't have too many of these!

If it is a serious injury, leave it to your doctor because they will certainly be better at offering advice and will recommend how long to have off exercising. Although this chapter may sound obvious, there are still so many people that forget to do the basis and it costs them later on. So, don't let that be you!

Training Tips

Not your average Joe can complete these circuits, meaning you can consider yourself a proper athlete if you consistently train HIIT Circuits. As an athlete, you will always have to be on top form because one day that you miss, because you "couldn't be bothered", can be the difference between success and failure. That may sound extreme for those of you who just have the goal to lower your body fat percentage, but you still must fully commit if you want your dream body. So, this leads me to suggest some training tips that will help you in the long run, each tip will be able to make a positive contribution towards helping you reach your fitness goal.

Glucose Before a Workout – When you are training as hard as you possible can, you will need as much energy as you can get. That leads me to suggest glucose. Glucose is a type of sugar (simple carbohydrate) found in many foods, although I suggest in the diet section to restrict the foods you consume that contain simple carbohydrates as the glucose that your body doesn't use is stored as fat, I suggest this for a pre workout meal/drink because you will be using up that glucose. As long as you get your glucose supply from something natural (no added sugar). A couple examples of having glucose before a HIIT Circuit include:

- Drinking a Lucozade 30 minutes before a HIIT Circuit.
- Having a handful of fruit 30 minutes before a HIIT circuit.

Glucose is a relatively healthy simple carbohydrate that can, as long as it is not consumed in large quantities, help you get the energy you need for the workout. Glycogen is stored after excess glucose is consumed, after a while that glycogen is turned into fat which will increase body fat percentage (specifically around the belly area). Muscles use glycogen for energy, so that is why when you need this for a workout.

Caffeine Before a Workout - Secondly, I suggest for you to drink a caffeinated drink like coffee or an energy drink around an hour before a workout. This is because caffeine increases the brains alertness and arousal levels which tricks the brain to think the workout is easier than it actually is. Caffeine gives your body a big energy boost around 15 to 60 minutes after consumption which will help your body cope to the training load. What I find best about a pre workout caffeinated drink is that caffeine can shift muscles to burn fat quicker, preserve the glycogen store and allow for the muscles to work for longer and harder before wearing out. A drink that contains roughly 100mg of caffeine will do the job, obviously if you don't like caffeinated drinks or your body has a bad reaction to caffeine, then avoid them.

Extra Salt – Please take this with caution. As HIIT Circuits are difficult it will make you sweat more and lose more fluid. Salt (sodium chloride) is lost throughout the day because it leaves the body through sweat and urine – meaning for those that drink lots of water and exercise hard, you will need more salt in their body. It is impossible for me to suggest how much salt for you to consume daily because everyone's body is different, the recommended amount of salt is less than 6 grams a day. I suggest for you to consume between 5 to 6 grams of salt a day. Cramps usually occur when you do not have enough salt and it is common to have more cramps when consistently training at a higher intensity. So, get all the salt you need to stop them cramps causing you trouble.

The Wim Hof Breathing Technique – I am always researching ways in which can be beneficial to help people reach their fitness goals. I came across this guy on YouTube, Wim Hof, he has his own breathing technique that helps him with all sorts of extreme things – this man once ran a marathon in a desert with no water! The idea of his breathing technique is for the lungs to intake more oxygen than is released over a certain period which makes your blood more alkaline and causes hypoxia. This breathing technique could be considered as meditation and comes with many benefits.

This breathing method has been tested by scientists for many years now on normal people, like yourself, to prove that Wim is not a superhuman and the results show that it can bring a few benefits such as: increased energy, better sleep, increased determination, improved sports performance, stronger immune system, faster recovery and greater cold tolerance to anyone that consistently uses the breathing technique.

The breathing technique consists of 30 quick deep breaths (in through your nose and out through your mouth), followed by a large inhale and exhale to which you will then hold your breath for as long as you can before having to inhale, after the final inhale you hold your breath for 15 seconds. You can repeat this method up to 3 times. I strongly suggest giving this a try and follow his guided breathing technique on YouTube as that makes it easier to follow. From personal experience, I can say this method helps relax me which is a positive because I find myself to be restless in the evening – relaxation is important for recovery and growth.

I don't want to take any credit from the main man Wim Hof, that's why if you are interested, I suggest you check out his YouTube video on how to follow the Breathing Technique and find out all the benefits that come with it. Just to point out, this isn't something that will change your life overnight but if you stick to 10 minutes a day of mediation, eventually you will notice the positive changes it makes to your life.

https://www.youtube.com/watch?v=tybOi4hjZFQ

Stretching – Although you will stretch before and after each HIIT Circuit or workout, I still suggest for you to stretch regularly. An example of stretching regularly is waking up every day and starting your day with 10 to 15 minutes of deep stretches to extend your range of motion. The benefits of regular stretching can be found in the list below. Before I get to the list, this is a good opportunity for those with slight injuries or knocks such as back pain, stiff joints or sprained ankles to relieve all that stress put on their body and get prepared for exercise. The benefits include:

- Increases Flexibility – crucial for overall health and helps with everyday activities.

- Increases range of motion – this will give you more freedom of movement.

- Increases blood flow to muscles – this will shorten your recovery time and reduces muscle soreness.

- Great for Stress Relief – when you experience emotional or physical stress then your muscles are tense, meaning regular stretching will reduce stress held in places like your neck, shoulders and upper back.

- Improves posture – good posture brings a number of benefits, the most common one being that it will reduce back pain.

Now, it is probably a good idea that you put this to the test although that can be quite hard if you don't know what stretches to do, not to worry because I include a few stretches that you can try out every day.

Standing Hamstring Stretch – Stretches your hamstrings. 1) Stand with feet slightly apart and knees slightly bent. 2) Slowly bend your body forwards at the hips and lower your head towards the floor. 3) Reach down as far as possible with your arms to feel the stretch in your hamstrings and hold that position for 30 seconds before slowly standing back up.

Seated Shoulder Squeeze – Stretches your deltoids and great for fixing posture. 1) Sit on the floor with knees bent and feet flat on the floor. 2) Take your arms behind your lower back and lock fingers. 3) Straighten and extend your arms to squeeze your shoulder blades together. Hold that for 3 seconds and continue to repeat that a few times.

Knee to Chest Stretch – Stretches your lower back and glutes. 1) Lay down on the floor facing the ceiling/sky and use your arms to hold your knees into your chest. 2) Keep your lower back on the floor and apply extra force to push your knees into your chest to feel the stretch – hold for 30 seconds.

Extended Puppy Pose – A great stretch for your back. 1) Start on your hands and knees but have your arms fully extended in front of you, keeping your palms planted to the floor. 2) Push your hips up and back towards your heels. 3) Push through your palms onto the floor and you should feel the stretch across your back and shoulders – hold for 30 seconds.

Butterfly Stretch – Great stretch for Hips. 1) Sit on the floor with a straight back, knees bent out to the side and soles of feet together. 2) Hold your ankles, engage your core and slowly lower your chest towards your feet. Also press your knees towards the floor, hold this stretch when you can feel it in your legs and back for 30 seconds. 3) Once stretched, slowly raise your body back to the starting position and repeat a couple times.

Seated Neck Release – Great stretch to relieve tension from your neck. 1) Sit with your back straight and chest lifted. 2) Roll your neck to the left so your left ear almost touches your left shoulder. 3) You can press down gently on your head to extend the stretch and hold this for 30 seconds before repeating on the right side.

There you have it, just a few of these stretches which will take up 10 minutes of your day will help you gain all the benefits previously listed. You can also use the stretches included in the warmups to help improve flexibility. Please check out this website to find more detailed explanations and picture examples for each stretch.

https://www.self.com/gallery/essential-stretches-slideshow

Finding Time

Many of us have busy lives, to which may make it hard for you to find time to complete these HIIT Circuits. Although one HIIT circuit will take up roughly 20-30 minutes of your time, it still can be hard to find this time for when you are tired, working, looking after somebody or whatever else it may be. Unfortunately, I am not going to let that from stopping you get your workout in.

Break your day up, everyone has 24 hours in a day, but some people manage to get so much more done that others in the same time period, Kevin Hart or Joe Rogan are great examples of people who manage this. You need 8 hours to sleep, which leaves roughly 16 hours for you to do all your day-to-day activities. It sounds like lots of time, but it can go quickly and before you even know it you have missed your workout and you are behind on your work. Fortunately for you, I have included a list of tips to help you increase your productivity:

Don't snooze – Before you go to bed set your alarm in a place where you will have to physically get out of bed to turn it off, because once you are up you will not be tempted to go back to sleep. Once you are up, you will have a fresh and longer day to look forward to because you have added 9, or 18, or 27 minutes to your day by getting up earlier than usual.

No daytime TV – First of all, what is on TV during the day that is worth watching? Because I don't think there is anything decent on TV until the evening, if you do like a certain program that's on during the day then just record it and watch it later. Use your day wisely to get things done and use the time to watch TV later in the day as a reward for getting it done.

Put your phone away — By this I don't mean for you to never touch your phone again, just put it away at times where you have stuff to do because it is a big distraction. For example, if you have an hour to get some work done, but you spend 20 minutes of that time scrolling on your phone then you have wasted 20 valuable minutes of work time, which will make you fall behind. It may be hard to concentrate for that entire hour, but once you hide the distractions like a phone, then you will find it much easier to crack out a solid hour of work and you may surprise yourself on how much you can get done.

Work when you work, rest when you rest — It's no-good dedicating the next hour of your day towards getting some work done if you are actually just going to spend 10 minutes on your phone, 10 minutes eating, 5 minutes watching videos and so on. You must stick to it, if you can get that solid hour of work done then you will free up more time for later in the day where you can kick your feet up and enjoy your rest – more importantly this will open up time for you to exercise!

Meal Prep – Cooking can take a while sometimes and leave you frustrated as you know you can use that time to do other things. That's why cooking in bulk for a few days will save you time later on in the week when you need it, as long as you have containers and space in your fridge you can cook meals for the future – just make sure to not prepare for too far in the future as food can go off!

Following these tips above should allow you to free up your time during the day, just freeing up a solid 30 minutes will allow you to get a great workout in. There is no better feeling than getting everything done in a day.

Goal Setting

You need a goal. Why you ask? Well because having a set goal gives you something to work towards and is a way for you to track your progress. You will need to set yourself smart goals. A smart goal should be:

Specific – This means for the goal to suit you. If you want to lower your body fat to 5% then write it down!

Measurable – This means that you can track your progress towards your goals. A goal to lower body fat is perfect because you can use Skinfold Calipers to measure your current body fat percentage to see if you are on target.

Attainable – The goals must be possible. If you set a goal that is way of out of reach within that time limit, then you may be putting lots of unwanted pressure on yourself to perform. This can lead to stress and disappointment for when you fall short of your goals.

Relevant – It must make sense. If you are looking to lower your body fat percentage, setting a goal to snap a pen in half makes absolutely no sense. Although I have taken that wrong example to an extreme, it still applies. Instead, your goal should be to lower your body fat percentage to 5%.

Time-bound – Your goals need a time limit towards it. Without a time-limit then it is less likely that you will reach your goals because there is no urgency for you to complete the goal.

The reason I say that you need to set Smart Goals, and not just a smart goal is because you should be setting 3 smart goals. They should be short-term, medium-term and long term. This puts you in a position where you will always have a goal to work towards, and once you reach your long-term goal then you will have to set another short-term, medium-term and long-term goal (even if that is to maintain your current body fat percentage) because that will keep you in a healthy routine. A short-term goal should have a time limit between a month and 3 months, medium term goal should be between 3 and 6 months while finally a long-term goal should be 9 months to a year.

If you don't know how to make your goals specific then think about what you want, if you want to look more toned/defined then your goal should be based on lowering body fat percentage (use skinfold calipers to measure progress). If your goal is based on looking bigger then focus on building lean muscle mass. If you goal is to become fitter over short distance events like sprinting, swimming or so on then use HIIT to increase your anaerobic endurance. Whatever your goal may be, simplify it and use the internet to search how you can measure your muscle mass, anaerobic capacity or whatever it may be.

Chapter 4 – How to Train Towards Completing HICT

When people have a goal of running a marathon, they don't just try to run it without any training because that is not the best idea. Unless you are God himself, then there is not a chance that you will be able to finish the marathon without training for it, because you have not given your body enough time to adapt to it. The same goes for HIIT Circuits. If you haven't exercised in a few months and you think that you will be able to complete a HIIT Circuit with no problem, then think again. I do not want to stop people trying a HIIT Circuit because they are too unfit to complete it, although yes, I understand that I have said this book is not for the beginners, they can still give It a go and train towards completing a HIIT Circuit.

Like I have repeated too many times throughout this book, I do not know the ability of everyone that is reading. So, if you don't know whether you can complete a HIIT Circuit or not, then try to complete the first HIIT Circuit in Chapter 6 and see how it goes. If you had to stop after a minute then no worries, you made a good attempt and I suggest looking at the previous books of this series so that you can get into a routine. If you completed over 50% of the circuit then well done, this book is good for you and you will be able to work towards completing it one day. If you managed to complete it relatively easily, then I suggest skipping this chapter – although that is quite stupid of me to say because the Circuits are in Chapter 6 and people don't usually read a book back to front... Anyway, maybe its best you refer back to this chapter after reading this book and completing a circuit.

Record

If you are at a stage where you can't complete the entire circuit, but you're not far off, then please don't give up because I am here to help you. After attempting a HIIT circuit it is important that you record what you have done. There are many things to record as there are many variables but below are the important variables to help you make progress.

Record the heart rate you were working at during the circuit. See if it was similar to the required Heart Rate listed on the Circuit. Record how long that you were exercising in the HIIT Circuit before having to stop to catch a breath. Finally, record any other things that happened while you were completing the circuit – if you needed a longer rest between exercises then note it down and so on.

Now that you have noted everything down, you will easily be able to see how far away you are from completing a HIIT Circuit. It is now up to you to set goals to improve certain aspects of your HIIT Circuit.

Example: For my first try at a HIIT Circuit I managed to follow the requirements for 10 minutes before having to come to a stop because I was out of breath. For the next time I train I want to try completing another 20 seconds of the HIIT Circuit before coming to a stop. I will continue to do this until I can fully complete the circuit. However, if I am able to complete another 20 seconds each HIIT Circuit session without being completely out of breath I will train for a bit longer until I have to stop.

Take-Action

Now it's your turn to take-action. The last subchapter suggests you record your results of the HIIT Circuit that you completed as a 'Test'. From those results you should be able to see a clear goal you have set yourself and it is now your turn to work towards them. Sticking with the previous example, you should complete the warmup then set up a timer for 10 minutes 20 seconds for when you next train the HIIT Circuit and aim to train until the timer finishes – you can even choose to carry on exercising for longer if you feel up to it. It is now your job to track your progress, so if you have trained an extra 30 seconds than the previous session, then note that down so you can aim to train for another 20 seconds past your personal best. Eventually, you will be at a stage where your goal to add an extra 20 seconds to each session will mean that you would have completed the entire HIIT circuit.

Unfortunately, taking action is easier said than done – but that doesn't mean it is not possible. You will need to self-motivate yourself to pick yourself up and train harder in each HIIT Circuit until you get to a stage where you can complete a HIIT Circuit from start to finish. It is more of a mental game from this point, the last Chapter in this book titled "Improvise, Adapt and Overcome" you will find plenty of motivational tips, advice on how to develop a determined mindset which will help you reach any goal you set yourself.

Improve

Progress is almost guaranteed to happen if you stick to a plan. The plan that includes a healthy diet and a consistent training routine with progressive overload will certainly let you improve to a stage where you can complete a HIIT Circuit. This is the fun part, where you can record your progress and feel proud of what you have achieved. Use your progress information to see if your goal can be achieved in a quicker period.

I suppose that you will be able to complete the HIIT Circuit after a while, and when you get to that stage, congratulations. You have reached your goal, but it shouldn't stop there. You should now introduce a variety of HIIT Circuits into your training routine, set yourself the 3 smart goals and keep pushing to improve. If you get to a stage where you feel you cannot set new goals as you don't feel the need to, then your goal should be to maintain your progress. Without maintaining, you will get back to a stage where you become unhealthy and struggle to complete a circuit.

Are you a Beginner?

I may have mentioned many times that this book isn't suitable for beginners, but if you are a beginner and want to give it a go, I am not going to stop you. This sub-chapter is just for any people who may be in a position where they haven't exercised for months, they don't know much about a healthy diet or a good exercise routine and the basics of keeping fit. It is completely fine if you are in this position because we all have to learn somehow.

People that get started with exercise are more likely to get injured because they don't know what they are doing, they try to rush things, or they have restrictions holding them back. Any restrictions like back pain, pain/stiffness in your joints, sprained ankles and so on all make the likelihood of you getting injured during exercising quite high, these restrictions can be formed over a lifetime. Luckily, these restrictions can be reversed with a number of methods so hopefully make exercising less painful and worthwhile for you in the future. In "Circuit Training for Beginners" you can find many gentle stretches, exercises and a recovery plan which will prepare your body slowly so you can start exercising safely.

Starting something new is always tough, especially when the workload is much higher than recommended. But don't let that discourage you, I am always here to support you. What to take from this: if you are a beginner then I suggest getting into a light exercise routine before tackling any of the HIIT Circuits. Slow and steady wins the race, so use the advice given in this chapter to work towards completing a HIIT Circuit.

Chapter 5 – The Warmups and Cooldowns for HICT

A very straight forward chapter that contains warmups and a cooldown. You should know how important it is to prepare for a workout by warming up beforehand, I am sure most people know this but either can't be bothered to do so or forget about it. It is also important to cool down after a workout, people are more likely to forget the cool down because they think they have completed the workout and want to get on with the rest of their day.

Warmups

Warmups are essential to carry out before training, the idea is to raise your heart rate and loosen the muscles you will use in the workout. You will need to raise your heart rate to around 70% to 80% of your max heart rate during the warmup to prepare for HIIT, this is so the right nutrients and oxygen is delivered to the muscles so they can perform at a high intensity. Without a warmup, it is highly likely you will suffer an injury.

Below you can find the heart raisers and stretches that make up "Warmup 3" and "Warmup 4". It comes clears that in this series the warmups and cooldowns are linked to the circuits later provided in this book. So, make sure you have a good look at the HIIT Circuits to see how they match up with the warmups, the harder HIIT Circuits are more likely to link to Warmup 4.

Warmup 3 (5 Minutes) –

- Light Jog on Spot – 1 minute
- Walking Knee Hugs – 30 seconds
- Sexy Circles – 30 seconds

- Arm Extension Hold – 30 seconds

- Ankle Rolls – 30 seconds

- Lateral Split Squat Stretch – 30 seconds

- High Kick Outs – 30 seconds

- Heel Flicks – 1 minute

Warmup 4 (5 Minutes)

- Light Jog – 1 minute

- Childs Pose – 30 seconds

- Calves Stretch – 30 seconds

- Hamstring Stretch – 30 seconds

- Chest Stretch – 30 seconds

- Side Lunge – 30 seconds

- Backpedaling – 30 seconds

- 5 Burpees (Do this in your own time)

Cooldowns

As explained before, cooldowns take place after a workout to allow gradual recovery by lowering the heart rate slowly. Stretches are certainly needed after a HIIT circuit as your muscles would be tighter after a high intensity session. Cooldowns should be slow, while including a range of stretches to increase the range of motion and light exercises to bring down the heart rate. Cooldowns typically last around 3 to 5 minutes. I will list a good cooldown to perform after a HIIT circuit:

Cooldown 3 (5 minutes)

- Light Jog on Spot – 60 seconds
- Lunges – 30 seconds
- Close the Gates – 30 seconds
- Seated Spinal Twists – 30 seconds
- Neck Rolls – 30 seconds
- Calf Raises – 30 seconds
- Bicep Stretch – 30 seconds
- Shake off Arms and Legs – 60 seconds

There is a reason why these are included in this book, that's because you will do a warmup before every HIIT Circuit and a Cooldown after every HIIT circuit. You cannot create shortcuts, if you think these aren't important then please don't complain when you get injured because the most common injuries are caused by skipping the warmup and cooldown. Although I may be sounding harsh, people don't always follow the basics and its costs them, I have always loved to take shortcuts, but it eventually caught up with me. Moral of the story: Don't cut corners!

Chapter 6 – The High Intensity Circuits to Burn Your Body Fat!

Here are the tough circuits I bet you cannot wait to smash through. There are five HIIT circuits that go up in difficulty. The five main circuits are titled "HIIT Circuit 1", "HIIT Circuit 2", "HIIT Circuit 3", "VHIIT" and "100%". Just like normal, all circuits are listed with all the exercises, the warm-ups and the cooldowns that link to them. You can find the warmup and cooldowns in Chapter 5 as well as find the exercise descriptions in Chapter 7.

As previously explained, HIIT stands for High Intensity Interval Training and VHIIT stands for Very High Intensity Interval Training – this should give the message that not everyone will be able to complete the circuits like planned. Although that doesn't mean you cannot have a go at them, just work to the requirements that are located above the circuit and do your best. If you came from the previous book and gave the HIIT taster a good go then you should be ready to include more HIIT circuits into your fitness routine.

I have tried my best to include a range of exercises for each HIIT Circuit so that you are working most muscle groups in the body – a whole body workout also provides great balance and won't leave you looking top heavy! Also check out the Abdominals HIIT Circuit, this is specific to training your core which helps burn belly fat.

What Makes HIIT Circuits Harder?

This short segment will provide you with enough information to make your own circuits. A standard circuit that you can find in my other two books and it is very similar to a HIIT circuit because it contains a list of exercises with a period of rest in-between. The main difference between HIIT Circuits and Normal Circuits is that the rest period of the normal circuits is equal to the time spent exercising the exercise while the rest period is either slightly longer, equal or shorter in HIIT circuits – this is because rest is much more appreciated after working at a high intensity, so starting off with a longer rest makes the HIIT Circuit easier and the rest time can be reduced to pose a real challenge. The main difference is the increased intensity, you will discover how tough it is to exercise above 80% of your max heart rate, with the normal circuits you would have been working at an intensity below 80% which is easier for your body to recover from.

HIIT Circuit 1

The first HIIT circuit of the book so that makes it the least challenging, although don't underestimate this circuit as it will still leave you sweating. This is the least difficult because it is the shortest to complete a set.

Complete 3 sets, Train in the Hard Training Zone (Around 80% of Max HR). Rest for 30 seconds between each exercise and rest for 2 minutes between sets. This circuit will take roughly take 25 minutes to complete including the warmup and cooldown.

Warmup 3

1. Burpees – 20 seconds
2. Bicycle Crunch – 20 seconds
3. Tuck Ups – 20 seconds
4. Shoulder Pushups – 20 seconds
5. Forward Kick Outs – 20 seconds

6. Open and Close Gates – 20 seconds

Cooldown 3

HIIT Circuit 2

Complete 2 sets, Train in the Hard Training Zone (Around 80% of Max HR). Rest for 30 seconds between each exercise and rest for 2 minutes between sets. This circuit will take just over 25 minutes to complete including the warmup and cooldown. This circuit includes more exercises to increase the variety of the circuit, I have also alternated the time spent on each exercise to increase the difficulty.

Warmup 3

1. Lying Superman Hold – 30 seconds

2. Fast Feet – 15 seconds

3. Wall sit – 30 seconds

4. Twist and Point – 15 seconds

5. Skipping – 30 seconds
6. Flutter Kicks – 15 seconds
7. Plank to Pushups – 30 seconds
8. Side Plank – 15 seconds a side

Cooldown 3

HIIT Circuit 3

Complete 2 sets, Train in the Hard Training Zone (Around 85% of Max HR). Rest for 20 seconds between each exercise and rest for 2 minutes between sets. This circuit will take just over 20 minutes to complete including the warmup and cooldown. Although this is shorter than the previous circuits, you are required to work hard.

Warmup 4
1. Twist and Point – 20 seconds
2. Snake Pushups – 20 seconds
3. Mountain Climbers – 20 seconds

4. Squat Jumps – 20 seconds

5. Standing Side Crunches – 20 seconds

6. Ali Shuffle – 20 seconds

7. Straight Punches – 20 seconds

8. Lunges and Twist – 20 seconds

9. Wall Sit – Hold 20 seconds

10. Twist Jumps – 20 seconds

Cooldown 3

VHIIT Circuit

Now it's time to move to the Maximum Training Zone, where the real gains are made. Your body may have not worked this hard in a very long time and to be honest, that's understandable.

Complete 3 sets, Train in the Maximum Training Zone (90% of Max HR). Rest for 30 seconds between each station and rest for 2 minutes between sets. This Circuit will take roughly 25 minutes to complete including the warmup and cooldown. Make sure to rest properly in the rest periods as you need all the energy you can get.

Warmup 4

1. Half Squat Jumps – 20 seconds
2. Power star – 20 seconds
3. Bicycle Crunches – 20 seconds
4. Mountain Climber – 20 seconds
5. Boxer Squats – 20 seconds
6. Fast High Knees – 30 seconds

Cooldown 3

100%

This one is mental, working at 100% of your heart rate is very hard to achieve but of course it is possible. As you are exercising as hard as you possibly can, the time spent on exercise will be short, but I will keep the rest periods short, so your heart rate doesn't drop dramatically.

Complete 2 sets, Train in the Maximum Training Zone (Work as hard as you can – 100% of Max HR). Rest for 20 seconds between exercises and 2 minutes between sets. Will take 20 minutes to complete including the warmup and cooldown. Do not attempt as a complete beginner. On your rests, I suggest sitting/standing upright with your hand behind your head to intake as much oxygen as possible.

Warmup 4

1. Fast Feet - 20 seconds
2. Burpees with Pushup – 20 seconds
3. Diamond Pushups - 20 seconds
4. Side Plank – 20 seconds
5. Reverse Crunches - 20 seconds
6. Squat Thrust – 20 seconds
7. Snake Pushups – As many as possible

Cooldown 3

If you are an absolute animal then you can make that circuit harder by adding more exercises, spending longer on each exercise. I managed to complete this circuit, but I was out of breath for ages afterwards. Feel free to share you experience within the Facebook group!

Abdominal HIIT Circuit

I had to throw this in, it was only right because everyone wants a nice, toned stomach or six-pack. This circuit targets your abdominals and obliques to help you look great in front of a mirror with a strong core. From my experience, I find that abdominal workouts where there is little rest between the exercises allow for better results because the gains are made while the core is engaged – this is the reason for the short rests.

Complete 3 sets, Train in the hard training zone (Around 80% of Max Heart Rate). Rest for 10 seconds between each exercise and 2 minutes between each set. This will take you roughly under 20 minutes to complete including the warmup and cooldown.

Warmup 3

1. Bicycle Crunch – 20 seconds
2. Flutter Kicks – 20 seconds
3. Mountain Climber – 20 seconds
4. Plank to Pushups – 20 seconds
5. Knees to Chest – 20 seconds
6. Side plank – 20 seconds each side

Cooldown 3

I have managed to complete all these circuits, although I do admit the 100% circuit is ridiculous, it is still possible. Don't forget that I have been training for years and if you can't complete it the first time don't give up because it takes mental strength to complete, you will have to work towards it and enjoy doing so. The resistant exercises like push-ups or squats may make you feel like you are working slower compared to completing the other exercises, don't worry about this because your body has a harder time when having to push/pull bodyweight which will maintain your high heart rate even when you think you are training slowly.

How Often to Train

If you have come from either of the previous two books, then you know that the recommended time for exercise is either 150 minutes of moderate physical activity or 75 minutes of vigorous activity.

You are now at a level where you should be way above the recommended time for exercise each week. I would suggest for those training at the top level to be training HIIT Circuits 6 or 7 days a week. For those working their way up towards completing a HIIT Circuit then I suggest training 4 days a week from the start and keep building up your workload until you reach 6 days a week. You can of course complete 3 days of HIIT and 4 days of weight training if you are looking to build up muscle quickly. There are so many ways you can include HIIT Circuits into your routine.

Make Your own HIIT Circuit

Below I will give you a template of how you can create your own circuit. I think it is important to give people the option to train the way that suits them. Feel free to use the exercises included from any of the books in this series, or any of your own exercises that you love. Most importantly, make it fun. Below is the list of variables that you must fill in to make up the Circuit.

Number of Sets:

Training Zone:

Rest Time Between Exercises:

Rest Time Between Sets:

Time of Complete Circuit:

Exercises Included:

1.

2.

3.

4.

Chapter 7 – Each Exercise With a Detailed Description and Photo

HIIT 1 Exercises

Burpee - Now this is a hard exercise to start with, but it is worth it. Start in the usual starting position. Then drop to the ground into a crouch position shown in the 1st photo with your hands planted on the ground. From the crouch position, stretch your legs out to a high plank position shown in the 2nd photo. Then you will want to hop your feet back into the first crouch position followed by a powerful jump upwards by pushing through your heels and hold your arms up to land like the 3rd photo shows (while in mid-air). You will then repeat all the above without resting for the time required. I recommend practising this exercise as you will want to be quick with this in the HIIT Circuits. Burpees are a whole-body workout meaning they build muscular strength and endurance in the upper and lower body.

Bicycle Crunches - Lay flat on the floor facing the ceiling with both hands behind your head. Keep your head and shoulders lifted off the ground for the entire activity by using your arms to slightly pull away from the floor. Start by bending your left knee towards your chest while your right leg is bent with your right foot on the floor, while you bend your left knee to your chest, twist your upper body and head to the left and you should feel it in your obliques (side abs). From that position, extend your left leg out forwards, twist your body from left to right using your lower back and bend your right knee towards your chest. Continue to swap legs and twist from left to right, right to left for the time provided. This exercise is best for burning fat around the abdominal area, while working the rectus abdominals, hips and obliques.

Knees to Chest – Lay on the floor facing the sky, with your legs fully extended. In one movement, bring your knees to your chest using your lower back and legs. Hold your legs in position (Photo 2) for a split second before relaxing your arms and pushing your legs back into the starting position (Photo 1). Continue to crunch your knees to and from your chest, this exercise is great for strengthening and defining your lower abs.

Shoulder Push-ups – Get into the position that the 1st photo shows, to do this plant hands on the floor so that they are in line with your shoulders, then place your tiptoes on the floor but stick your bum up and close the distance between your hands and feet. To do a shoulder push-up, keep your hands and toes planted and use your arms to lower your face near the ground, once you reach a stage where you can't go down any further push back using your arms. This mainly works your deltoids, making you work your shoulders as well as working chest and triceps.

Forward Kick Outs – Stand on the spot keeping on your toes. Then simply just raise your left knee while keeping it bent (Kung-Fu Stance photo 1), after it is lifted maintain balance and in one motion you should kick out your left lower leg and bring it back in to the "Kung-Fu" stance. Lower your left foot to the ground and repeat with your right leg. This may not be the most intense exercise, but it improves balance, and it can be done quickly so that you will feel the burn at the end of a circuit.

Open and Close the gates – A relatively gentle exercise for HIIT. Begin by standing up straight with your feet moderately apart, then lift your left knee up in front of you, move your leg roughly 90 degrees to the left by rotating your hip (keep foot off the ground). Now that you have opened the gate, you need to close the gate, do this by moving your left knee 90 degrees right then lowering your foot to the ground (Just reverse your movements from opening the gate). Repeat that on your right leg but rotate to the right instead of left when opening the gate. Great exercise for improving balance it also will work glutes, hamstrings and keep your hips loose.

HIIT 2 Exercises

Lying Superman Hold – Starting position: Picture 1 shows that you should lay down facing the floor with your arms slightly in front of you and your legs slightly apart while relaxed. Use your core and lower back to raise your arms and legs off the ground, hold this position for a split second before relaxing your muscles back into the starting position. Continue this for the time given, a great core exercise while working lower back and upper legs. Complete this as quick as you can to maintain the high heart rate.

Fast Feet – Start standing with feet wider apart than usual and knees slightly bent. This is a fast-paced exercise so go through it slowly before picking up the pace. Keep your knees slightly bent and lift your left foot slightly off the ground (about an inch or so), then lower your left foot to the ground while simultaneously lifting your right foot off the ground. Keep alternating feet and do this at a fast pace. This exercise should wear you out and shoot your heart rate up – meaning you will burn fat. This may feel like sprinting on the spot.

Wall Sit – This requires space in front of a wall. Start by standing with your back to the wall, squat down and sit with your back against the wall like the photos show below. Hold this position for the time given and you will certainly feel this in your glutes, calves and quads. After the previous exercises, the wall sit will hurt even more, it is all about mental toughness to get through it.

Twist and Point – Begin with hands and feet on the floor just like the press-up position. Then lift your left hand off the ground and twist your torso to face to the left so that your right hand is holding you up, while in that position raise your left hand as high as you can before bringing your hand back down to the ground to balance the weight of your body onto both arms. Then repeat this on your right side by holding your body up with your left hand and have your right arm is pointing up. Continue to switch between arms for the time period. This exercise will allow you to build endurance and strength in your triceps, shoulders and pectorals. Other muscles trained: upper back muscles and abdominals.

Skipping – This does not require a jump/skipping rope however if you have one you may as well use it. If you have the rope, then skip just like how you usually would – try to skip quickly and switch feet if you are skilled. If you do not have a rope then no worries, pretend that you are holding a rope and then skip – you may look slightly silly, but this exercise is still effective for burning calories and improves your foot-eye coordination. If you are pretending to skip, then do this at a face pace to keep your Heart Rate high.

Flutter Kicks - Lay on the floor facing the sky with your hands behind your head - lifting your head and shoulder off the floor. Keep your legs straight and lift your left leg up while keeping your right leg slightly off the ground. From that position lower your left leg to the hovering position and raise your right leg up slightly like the second photo shows. Continue to move between the positions shown in the two photos below. This exercise is brilliant for strengthening back muscles, lower rectus abdominals and hip flexors. Don't let your feet touch the floor!

Plank to Push up – Start in the usual push-up position on your hands and tiptoes. From the push up position place your left forearm on the floor followed by your right forearm, do this while keeping your feet in the same position. Then as soon as your right forearm is placed on the floor you will be in the plank position. From this plank position get back into the push-up position by placing your left palm on the ground, then your right palm and finally push up with your arms. Continue to move from the two positions shown in the photos below. This exercise is great for building strength and endurance in your deltoids, pectorals, triceps and your rectus abdominals.

Side Plank – Start by laying down with your left forearm on the floor with the side of your left foot on the floor, look at the 1st photo for inspiration. Hold this position for the time given in the HIIT Circuit instructions before swapping to the right side. For the right-side plank, place your right forearm on the ground and the right side of your right foot on the ground while keeping your body off the floor (2nd photo). This exercise works your obliques and should make most of your body ache as it is the last exercise of the circuit.

HIIT 3 Exercises

Twist and point – Previously Explained. Make sure you complete quicker reps to maintain the higher heart rate.

Snake Push-ups – These are brutal! Start in a high push-up position (photo 1), tiptoes on the floor with legs slightly bent, bum sticking up and your hands planted on the floor shoulder width apart. To complete a Snake Push-up: use your arms to lower your chest to the ground while simultaneously moving your chest slightly forwards to get to the position of photo 2. Then from that position push up through your arms to get to the final position where you should be ready to go again. This exercise is great for triceps, deltoids and pectorals, the angle at which you push up causes your muscles to exert more.

Mountain Climbers - Start with your hands and feet on the floor like you're in a push up position. Then while keeping your hands planted on the ground, bring your left knee to your chest. From this position (Photo 1), kick your left leg back to where it was in the push up position, while at the same time bringing your right knee to your chest. Continue to switch from the positions shown in both pictures below. Great exercise specific to burning belly fat.

Squat Jumps – Firstly stand with your feet slightly wider than shoulder width apart and facing outwards. Then squat down by sitting back, shifting your weight into your heels while bending your knees, once you get as low down as you can, push up through your heels and toes to jump up explosively. Use your arms to help create momentum for your jump. Once you land the squat jump you should carry on squatting down and jumping up until your times up! Great for building strength mainly in quads, hamstrings, calves, glutes as well as lower back muscles and abdominals. Requires many different muscles to perform a jump meaning you will burn calories and improve explosive power. Try to get as many jumps as you can in the time provided.

Standing Side Crunch – Begin by standing straight with your hands behind your head with fingers locked together. Use your hands to push your head down to the left while leaning to the left and raising your left knee (2nd photo), this should make you feel a slight burn in your obliques. Hold that position for a split second before lowering your left leg. Then lean to the right and raise your right knee to feel the same burn just this time on the other side (3rd photo). This exercise helps your improve balance and strengthen obliques. Complete quicker than usual to match the required heart rate.

Ali Shuffle – Start with your left foot in front of your right and knees slightly bent (1st photo). Then hop off the ground slightly so you can bring your left foot back and your right foot forwards at the same time (2nd photo), when you land you should hop again straightaway and then shuffle your feet back to the starting position. Do this continuously so you are always swapping feet. A great cardiovascular activity that will improve foot-eye coordination and will give you fast feet. (If you have ankle weights knocking about then stick them on!) This exercise was made popular by the great Muhammad Ali and look how it helped him out. Get as many shuffles in as you can in the time given.

Straight Punches – Start by standing in a causal boxing stance, do this by placing your weak foot (pointing forwards) in front of your strong foot (which should face outwards) and hold your arms high with your fists clenched like the 1st photo shows below – always keep your knees slightly bent. To throw a left straight punch then simply extend your left arm out quickly until you cannot extend your arm anymore, which then you should instantly bring your arm back to the starting position – always keep a clenched fist and the punch should be like a snap. To throw a right straight punch, follow the same steps as the left straight punch but twist your body into the punch. My boxing book can always help you with form. The benefits from this include faster hands, will make you sweat and potentially hand eye coordination. Repeat left-right-left-right straight punches very quickly for the time period.

Lunges with Twists- From a standing position take one foot forward and keep the other foot planted, shift your weight onto the front leg and bend both legs. Once in the lunge position twist

172

your body to the left (Picture 1) then to the right (Picture 2) using your arms and lower back then finally step back into a standing position. Works your legs and lower back. Also, remember to alternate the leg which you lunge froward with.

Wall Sits – Previously explained. Will be harder in this circuit due to the higher intensity causing your muscles to ache more, you sure will have strong legs if you stick to this.

Twist Jumps – Stand with feet slightly wider than shoulder width apart, drop into a squat while twisting your body and arms to the left. Then quickly swing your arms to the right to and use your lower back to twist your torso to the right while jumping up through your heels, so that you jump up and rotate 90 degrees clockwise in the air. Land the jump and repeat, change direction whenever you feel like it. Improves agility, flexibility in hips and leg strength. Complete quickly, get as many jumps in as possible.

VHIIT Exercises

Half Squat Jumps – Start in the position shown in the first photo, to do this place your feet shoulder-width apart and slightly bend your legs. From this position bend your knees a little bit to drop down into the half squat, then spring up through your heels to elevate slightly off the ground (Photo 2). Land from the jump in the position of photo 1, and you are good to repeat again and again. This exercise is great for getting a sweat on and also strengthens legs. These need to be performed very quickly, don't jump too high so you can get as many jumps as possible in the time.

Power Star – This is like an explosive star jump. Start by standing with legs together, then bend your knees to bend down and touch your toes (1st photo), before quickly jumping straight up and raising your arms with side of you to appear as a star (Blurry 2nd Photo). On the way back down to the floor bring your arms back to your sides and legs together so you are ready to do another Power Star. Another great cardio exercise which mainly works the leg muscles, but is an entire body workout.

Bicycle Crunches – Previously Explained. Work faster.

Mountain Climbers – Previously Explained. Work Faster.

Boxer Squat – Begin by standing with feet facing slightly outwards and placed wider than shoulder width apart. Keep your hands up in a boxer guard (1st photo). Squat down by sitting back and bending your knees as far down as you can go. Then from the squat position push up through your heels back to the starting position and throw a straight left and a straight right punch (1-2). To punch, fully extend your arms your quickly in front of you one after the other then bring your arms back to the starting boxer guard position to go again. Remember to be quick!

Fast High Knees – Start by standing in usual position but try to keep light on your feet. This needs to be fast paced: Firstly, lift your left knee as high as you can (1st photo), then lower your left foot to the ground while you raise your right knee as high as you can (2nd photo). Repeat this very quickly throughout

the 30 seconds, it may feel like sprinting on the spot.
Great cardio and will certainly burn many calories.

100%

    Fast Feet - Previously explained, just now
needs to be as fast as you possibly can.

    Burpee with Push-up – Prepare yourself to
do a burpee (previously explained), carry out the
burpee but this time when you drop down into the
push-up position instead of hopping your feet closer
to your hands to get back up, you should complete

a push-up by lowering your chest to the ground and pushing back up with your arms (Transition from photo 2 to photo 3). After you complete the push-up then you can bring your feet to your hands to jump up. Try to be quick with the push up to maintain high Heart Rate.

Diamond Push-up – A very tough push-up indeed. Start with hands and feet on the floor like how you would usually start for many floor exercises, however, bring your hands closer together and into a diamond shape like the first photo shows below. Always keep your hands and feet planted to the ground while you use your arms to lower your chest to your hands, from that position (photo 2) push back up with your arms. This kind of push-up is great for strengthening triceps, also strengthens pectorals and deltoids.

Side Plank – Previously explained, will be harder due to higher intensity of other exercises.

Reverse Crunches – Lay flat on your back facing the ceiling/sky to get into the starting position. Always keep your hands planted on the floor either side of you for support. Then bring your knees as far as possible towards your face while keeping your feet together (Photo 1). When your knees are near your chest, extend your legs forwards while keeping them off the floor (Photo 2). Continue to switch between these two positions below using your core and lower back to move your legs. This exercise works the full length of the rectus abdominal muscle, making this the most efficient exercise for getting a six-pack.

Squat Thrusts – Start with hands and feet on the floor like in a high push up position (1st Photo). Remember to always keep your hands planted in the same position and hop both your feet together forwards and back repeatedly (Photo 2 to Photo 1), when hopping forwards aim to bring your knees close to your chest and when you hop back just get into the starting position. Try to take most of your bodyweight with your arms. This exercise is brilliant for burning belly fat.

Snake Push-ups – Previously explained. You will have to give it everything for this exercise, I imagine that you will be absolutely shattered but you have to keep going.

Warmup Exercise Descriptions

Jog on Spot – Not much to say, just like you are running but not in any direction.

Knee Hugs – From a standing position, raise your left knee to your chest and hold it for a few seconds before letting go and swapping to perform the hug with your right leg.

Sexy Circles – Stand tall with your feet wide apart and keep your hands on your hips. For the 30 seconds, proceed to rotate your hips in circles using your legs and lower back to do so. This exercise loosens up your hips and groin, remember to spend

15 seconds going clockwise, 15 seconds anti-clockwise and make sure you look good doing it!

Arm Extension Hold – In a standing or sitting position, raise both arms up as high as you can (so that your palms are facing up) and lock your fingers together. From that position roll your shoulders up to extend your arms further and push up through your fingers, hold this for 10-15 seconds to give your arms a good stretch then you should stretch again after a slight rest. Overall, stretch twice in the 30 second period.

Ankle Rolls – Stand with feet shoulder width apart. Raise your left heel so that your tiptoes are on the floor and have your right foot planted on the floor, then rotate your left ankle clockwise using your tiptoes. After 15 or so seconds, switch foot so your right foot is on its tiptoes then rotate that for 15 seconds. This stretches the ligaments, muscles and tendons in and around your ankle.

Lateral Split Squat Stretch – Start by standing in a wide stance with your feet flat and your toes pointing straight ahead. Squat down towards the left while bending your left leg and keeping your right leg straight, hold this for 10-15 seconds before standing up and bending to the right to stretch your alternative leg. This stretches most of the major leg muscles and should be done slowly.

High Kick Outs – This requires plenty of space to complete. From a standing position you will need to kick out in front of you with your left leg while your right foot is planted, try to get your left leg as high as you can while keeping it extended. Once your foot gets as high as possible, bring your left leg down and repeat the kick out with your right leg. Continue to kick and swap legs for the 30 seconds. This yet again stretches leg muscles and uses your core.

Heel Flicks – From a standing position, kick your left foot back towards your bum while keeping your right foot on it tiptoes. Then as you bring your left foot down towards the floor you should kick back your right foot towards your bum. Continue to flick your feet towards your bum in the order of left foot, then right foot for a minute. This will loosen up your leg muscles and get your heart beating quicker.

Child Pose – Start by kneeling on the floor. From that position place both hands on the floor in front of you and continue to stretch your arms out as far as they can go. Eventually you will get to a point where you can't extend your arms any further, hold that position for 10 seconds before relaxing and going back to the kneeling position. Repeat that twice in the 30 second period to stretch your lower back.

Calves Stretch – Find a wall with a bit of open space in front of it. Stand in front of the wall and place your left foot on the wall, press down on the wall with your left tiptoes to stretch your calf, you should feel this burning sensation if you are doing it correctly. Hold that for 10 to 15 seconds before stretching your right calf.

Hamstring Stretch - To stretch your left leg: Start by standing up straight, then bend your right knee slightly while extending your left leg so your left heel is on the floor and your toes are pointing upwards. Hold this stretch for 10-15 seconds. Then switch leg by repeating the steps but alternatively. If you don't feel anything the press down with your hands onto your bent knee as this force will certainly stretch the hamstrings.

Chest Stretch – This can be done standing or sitting. Puff your chest out by inhaling heavily, then keep your arms behind your back. Your arms behind your back should be crossed and you need to try to touch your right elbow with your left hand and your left elbow with your right hand, as you are reaching your arms across, you will be stretching your chest. Hold the stretch for 10 seconds before having a break and going again.

Side Lunge – Begin by standing with feet shoulder width apart. Twist your left foot 90 degrees anticlockwise then lunge forwards in that direction while keeping your right foot planted. Hold that lunge for 10 to 15 seconds before stepping back in and rotating your left foot back to the starting position. Remember to do both sides by rotating your right foot 90 degrees clockwise then lunging forwards in that direction.

Backpedalling – As I understand many of you will be working out in a limited space, here is an alternative method on how to complete. From a standing position jog forwards a couple of steps, after that you will want to bend your knees and get low to run backwards around 4 steps (face the same direction just run backwards). Without sounding too crazy, you will continue to run back and forth for the time given.

5 Burpees – Previously explained. Just do 5 burpees in your own time as the final heart raiser before getting into the workout. Should take from 30 to 60 seconds, don't complete these burpees too quickly as it's a warmup.

Cooldown Exercise Descriptions

Light Jog on Spot - Just a slow gentle jog to lower your heart rate, which I imagine is pounding out of your chest after a HIIT Circuit.

Lunges – This is like the exercise "Lunges and Twist", without the twist. So, for this cooldown activity, lunge forwards with your left leg from a standing position and hold that lunge for 10 to 15 seconds before stepping back. Then lunge forwards with your right foot and hold for the remaining time. This will stretch the major leg muscles and lower back.

Close the Gates – Open and Close the Gates previously explained in this chapter. You will just need to complete the second part of that exercise, for example you will start with your left knee raised 90 degrees to the left to which you will use your hip to rotate your knee clockwise until it is directly in front of you. Make sure to close the gates slowly to increase the range of motion on your hips. Also remember to close the gate for both legs.

Seated Spinal Twists – Begin by sitting down with your back straight. For the 30 seconds you will need to slowly rotate your body from left to right using your lower back and arms.

Neck Rolls – A very nice dynamic stretch. Can be done standing or sitting. Roll your head clockwise around your shoulders using your neck very slowly for 15 seconds, then roll your head anticlockwise for the remaining time.

Calf Raises – Start in the usual standing position but be on your tiptoes. Simply press up through your tiptoes slowly as high as you can go, once you reach that position slowly lower your heels to the floor. Continue to repeat that motion slowly to feel the burning sensation in your lower legs.

Bicep Stretch – To do this simply stretch out your left arm with the palm facing up. With your right hand, you should push down on the palm of the stretched-out arm. You should feel your forearm and bicep being stretched. Repeat on the other arm.

Shake off Arms and Legs – It is what it says. Spend a few seconds shaking your left leg off with your foot off the ground to increase blood flow, the do the same with your right leg. Keep both your arms down and shake them off gently for the time being as well. Not much else to say apart from give them a good shake.

Benefits of Training Muscles

Throughout this chapter, I have included the muscles that are worked during each exercise (for most of them at least). For most people that may not mean anything, so here is a section to explain why training each particular muscle is important and can help you in many ways.

Calf – This is the muscle that is found at the back of the leg below the knee, made up of two smaller muscles: Soleus and Gastrocnemius. This is a major leg muscle which supports your upper legs and body. Exercises that require for the calf to be used will make the calf stronger over time. Having strong calves is great because it allows for you to run faster, run for longer, jump higher, keep a more consistent running pace and can easily support your body if the rest of your muscles become heavier.

Quadriceps – These are located at the front of the leg above the knee. You engage your quads for most of the day, whether that's by walking or standing or biking then you will be using your quads, so they are important as they keep you moving. Having strong and flexible quads will boost your knee function because it will take most the stress away from the knees, your knees without any other muscular support are more likely to be damaged under stress from body weight (having weak quads is likely to end up knee osteoporosis). Having strong and flexible quads will also make daily activities like walking, running and standing easier for your entire body.

Hamstrings – These are tendons that are at the back of the thigh that attach the thigh muscle to the bone. This muscle is usually engaged during activities that involve bending the knee, for example: running, jumping or climbing. Stronger Hamstrings will allow you to achieve better speed, power and agility with exercise and many sports. Plus, having weak hamstrings will damage your knees. It is important to stretch your hamstrings out at the end of a workout because that will prevent them shortening and losing elasticity. Having strong hamstrings will also reduce strain on other ligaments or tendons, which reduces injury.

Glutes – The glutes are found in the buttocks and are considered one of the strongest muscles in the body. The benefits of having strong glutes include increased athletic performance as you can run faster, jump higher and become more agile. Also helps with injury prevention because strong glutes will reduce the strain on the lower back muscles, knees and leg muscles. Overall, having strong glutes will keep your body functioning to the best of its ability.

Biceps – Biceps are found in the front of your upper arm. The advantages of having strong biceps include improved bone density, a higher resistance to injury, greater upper body strength, bigger arms and will help you achieve more power in sports that involve throwing, tossing or swinging. Although biceps are difficult to engage without equipment, it still can be done.

Triceps – Found along the back of the upper arms. They allow for movement in your shoulders and elbows. Triceps are engaged when we straighten or lock our elbows – an example of this is by pushing objects away from us or exercises like push ups. Having strong triceps will help build upper body strength, which is helpful for stabilizing your shoulders, will increase your pushing power, will allow you to build larger arms which may make you appear more attractive. String Triceps will also help you with many sports and activities like tennis.

Pectoral – Located in the chest and is made up of four muscles. These muscles are commonly known as 'pecs', the pecs connect the front of the of the chest with the bones of the upper arms and shoulders. The pectoral muscles are used to move the arms and also moves the ribcage during deep breathing. Having strong pectoral muscles brings many benefits like:

- Can improve posture.
- Increases the strength in your back muscles – the back muscles are later explained.
- Increases upper body strength.
- Improving your ability to push things.
- Can improve your ability to perform swinging movements.
- Finally, it can allow for an improved appearance of the chest.

Shoulders – The deltoid muscles are the muscles that form the rounded contour of the shoulder. Having strong shoulders will make arm movements easier like throwing, tossing, pulling or pushing. It also helps with injury prevention, if you have weak shoulders but like to train pecs and triceps, then your shoulders are likely to get injured because the deltoids won't be able to cope with the workload that the other two muscles can handle. Of course, there is an appearance factor, it is likely that you will appear more attractive with bigger and wider shoulders.

Upper Back – Many muscles are involved in the upper back. There is not much point of me listing all the muscles, but you may have heard of lats, traps and rhomboids. Each muscle in your upper back has a job to keep the body held upright and allow for trunk movements. Below you can find a list of benefits that come with a strong upper back:

- Prevents injury as the back muscles take the stress away from the shoulders.
- Improves upper body strength – will allow you to pull heavier objects towards you.
- Increased support for neck and shoulders which will reduce potential neck and back pain.
- Helps maintain a good posture.
- Back muscles are the second strongest muscle group in the body, training those muscles expands plenty of energy which helps your body maintain high energy levels.
- Strong backs look good. (A common feature with all muscles)

Lower Back – Many muscles make up the lower back. Just like the upper back there is no point listing all the individual muscles but they allow us to stand and lift objects up. The benefits of a strong back are almost identical to the benefits that come with a strong upper back. The only differences being that strong lower back muscles can strengthen the core, leg and arm muscles.

I want this book to give you as much information as possible and I hope the information provided on the benefits that come with strengthening each muscle will encourage you to include more HIIT Circuits in your training routine. The most common benefit of building up all these muscles is that you will become a stronger, faster, and bigger individual. If you are starting off overweight, then don't think that building lean muscle will make you go up a size because you will just be building your perfect physique for when you do burn all the fat surrounding it. Building lean muscle mass has a huge correlation with injury prevention.

Plus, for you ladies that think building muscle will make you unattractive, don't stress about it because these exercises are hardly going to make you look masculine overnight and it's not a bad thing to be strong. Lean muscle mass will keep you looking toned and brings you all the benefits, so it's not something to miss out on.

Chapter 8 – Improvise, Adapt and Overcome

As I am sure you are all aware, 2020 has been unpredictable to say the least. With all the unfortunate events that have occurred, many people had to change the way they live – the most common difference being that many people have spent much longer inside. While most people just accept the change that they're not happy with or bored of, some people decide to improvise, adapt and overcome the change.

By that phrase I mean that people use their creativity to try carry on their normal life from home so that they are not wasting any valuable time, because you do only have one life at the end of the day which makes our time precious. This chapter is focused on mindset more than anything, providing lots of motivation to help you find your inner determination to get things done! Yes, I agree that relaxing at home for a couple days is nice, but for a month? Is that not boring? Just watching the same crap over and over again while making no progress towards any of your goals, because I'd say that is a terrible use of time.

I want this chapter not to only help you mentally to reach your fitness goals, but just you help you out generally. Mental health is a big concern worldwide and the problems caused by lockdown and isolation are putting people in a bad place. Being stuck inside with a lack of entertainment, facing loneliness or having no access to gyms really isn't great for your mental wellbeing. I want you to be able to look back at this lockdown period, or even if you are reading this in 2030, I want you to look back at a hard time in your life and feel proud of how you dealt with it.

Improvise

Instead of accepting that you can't do something because you find it too hard or there are restrictions holding you back, you have to break down the problem bit by bit to discover what is that is specifically causing you the problem. For example, with getting into a training routine it may be that you cannot wake up early in the morning to complete your workout – it is now your job to think about why you cannot wake up early. Is it because you went to be too late the night before? Is it because you can't find the motivation to get out of bed in the morning? Or it may be a little thing, did you forget to set an alarm?

Once you ask yourself these questions you may then realise why you can't do it. This improvising step is about finding where the problem lies and will hopefully show you what you can do to solve the problem in a way that is specific to you. Your problem won't be solved if somebody just says, "Well just wake up and get out of bed earlier". It is better if somebody asks you those questions and uses your answers to suggest solutions such as: "Remember to set an alarm for when you want to wake up", "Try to get to sleep earlier the night before", "C'mon, you need to get up because if you don't then you will not reach your goal". Of course, it is easier said than done, doing something about it has a much bigger impact towards reaching greatness.

The problem and solution there is quite concise, and I know that there are many other reasons why it is a struggle to get into a training routine. But that doesn't mean this method won't work for your problems or difficulties.

Now, it is most likely that you are going to be the only person asking yourself these questions and answering yourself, which may seem a bit crazy, but stay with me. It is much easier to feel motivated by having a PT or person there persuading you to get stuff done, but as it is likely you will be on this journey alone so that is why you must learn to motivate yourself. You will be the only person to ask yourself the questions on why you failed and come up with solutions on how to win.

Plus, there are many solutions for each problem, it's all about thinking outside the box. If you really don't like the idea of waking up early to complete a HIIT circuit, then you don't have to. Instead, you can complete the HIIT Circuit later on in the day, as long as you have a plan that works for you so that you don't have to make any sacrifices like waking up early. Please note this may result in other issues, but I am hoping you'll learn how to overcome them with this guide.

Adapt

This is the next stage of the mental mindset to go with fitness or anything really. I would like to say that this stage is where you go for it, this is where you make your first mark towards greatness. This may be the hardest step out of the three.

Sticking with the previous example which was all about not being able to wake up early enough to exercise, to adapt to solving the problem you would have to start making changes to what you do. For example, you would want to set alarm, go to bed earlier the night before and force yourself out of bed. That's the hardest part because once you are out of bed your body will get out of that resting state, all it leaves you to do now is complete the exercise and get on with the rest of your day. I use this example because it was something I previously struggled with, I found that in order to wake up earlier I had to leave my phone halfway across my room, so I had to physically get out of bed to click snooze – once I was up, there was no point me going back to sleep and that's how I got through my day.

You may find that the first time you do that something different to overcome your problem that the rest of your day may be much more difficult than imagined– for example if you exercise early in the morning for the first time you may find yourself struggling more to complete the exercise. This is because you are not used to the change as of yet and the overcome stage is what will help you bypass the struggle, the only way to get around this to keep going again and again. You may start to see that overtime it gets easier and it will be worth it in the long run. You can apply the adapt method to anything. You need to give your body time to adjust, it doesn't all happen overnight!

Overcome

The final step, the one that is achieved by consistency. The definition of overcome is when you succeed in dealing with (a problem or difficulty). You will reach the stage of overcoming once you are in a position when the thing that was stopping you reach your goal (for example not being able to wake up in the morning to exercise), is no longer a problem, just instead something that you complete comfortably (now being able to wake up on time every day and being prepared for the workout).

You can overcome any personal problem, but it is important that you stick to a routine to do so. The longer that you put off dealing with a challenge the harder it gets each day to build up courage/motivation to tackle that same challenge – in other words the longer you spend hesitating the more likely you are to give up. Giving up isn't an option, it doesn't let you achieve anything apart from regret.

In order to overcome your problem(s), you must follow the previous two steps "Improvise" – to discover what is causing your problem and how to get around it, "Adapt" – to start trying the method to get around the problem and now finally you must "Overcome" – to consistently get around the problem until eventually it is no longer a problem. To explain this, I will stick with the example of not waking up on time to train. To overcome this situation then you will want to do all you can to make sure that you wake up on time. This can be done by setting an alarm for when you want to wake up, by going to sleep earlier the night before and pushing yourself mentally to get up. If you get into a habit of following them 3 solutions, then eventually it will all become natural, after a while it won't even cross your mind that you are waking up earlier to exercise because your body clock will adapt to the new training time and you will feel great about yourself.

So, the best way to put it is that if you want to succeed then you will need to find something that works and stick to it. I am unaware of what is stopping you exercise or any of your other problems, that's why I hope for this to help you find your own solutions to your problems. I believe you can use this advice for any challenges you face, it seriously helps and is quite simple. You see many motivational tips for fitness which involve all these complications, but this simple technique will prevent you wasting time and feeling down.

If this doesn't help you overcome your problems to do with fitness, then you should probably look for personal trainers as support — there is only so much that I can write in this book and by email. I physically cannot be there to support you, that is why I want to point you in the direction of where to reach support because I want the best for you. There are many Fitness groups on Facebook you can join, or you can even contact your local gym to get into contact with a PT.

Short term Discomfort, Long term Gain

Living comfortably is a real privilege that many people get to experience every day, let's be honest most of us (including myself) take living comfortably for granted. It is only when we go through a period of stress or discomfort that we wish that we could go back to how we were living beforehand. But many people across the world don't live comfortably, which is a huge problem, but sadly it is just how it is and will take years to sort out. Although, there is limit to how I can help people in discomfort (donation is my best option), this makes me think about how people that live in struggle are generally more driven and are mentally prepared for anything that comes their way. You often hear these 'Rags to Riches' stories about people who had absolutely nothing and worked their ass off to get to the top – Manny Pacquiao is a great example.

I am not saying that you should ditch your comfortable life just to increase your chances of becoming successful. But instead, you should consider putting your body/mind in a short period of discomfort. Why? This is because discomfort to the mind or body is something that we are not used to, this makes your body or mind slowly adapt to the change which then allows for growth. You ever heard of the term, no pain no gain? This saying is exactly what discomfort will bring you, that short period of physical or mental pain will make you physically and mentally stronger in the future.

There are endless ways on how you can get into a position of discomfort, whether that is staying for an extra hour of work, running an extra mile, or waking up earlier each week. Each method of discomfort will make you grow towards your goals and of course I will use fitness to prove this. So, if you really want to reach your goals, you have to sacrifice your comfort for it. I think that is a fair deal because a period of discomfort every now and then will help you develop a strong mindset to hit any target you set yourself.

You must think long term. I understand it is hard to turn down short term comfort, like a glass of wine or a chocolate bar, because it is nice. Remember that a chocolate bar will do absolutely no good for you and you know that, but if you stick to your healthy diet then in the long run you will achieve your fitness goal and you don't have to completely cut out nice unhealthy food – just limit it to once a week and stick to the limits.

Living comfortably is likely to make you lazy, unmotivated and you will not make progress to life towards your goals. Unless your goal is to be a couch potato! So, look for periods of short-term discomfort, it will do you some good.

Short term discomfort links to progressive overload in a way that you are pushing your body harder during exercise to make that fitness gain over time. But this chapter doesn't always have to help you with fitness, whether you find talking to new people uncomfortable, whether you are scared to put your name out there or whatever the reason is, you should just get it done. It may be embarrassing or wrong at first, causing discomfort, however you will learn from mistakes and come back better and more confident. I believe confidence to be the best driving factor to help to reach your goals, and you can build your confidence through short term discomfort!

Exercise is Good for Your Brain

The physical benefits of exercise are easier to spot and have already been discussed. Although the physical benefits are nice, I believe the mental benefits to massively outweigh the physical benefits. I love to exercise because I feel great afterwards, I would never have known why I feel so good after a workout without research. Below is a list of mental benefits exercise can bring:

- Physical Activity increases the endorphin levels – endorphins are the 'Happy' chemicals in the brain which make you feel great. This mood booster can decrease the symptoms of depression and anxiety.

- Decreased Stress – Increasing your heart rate over a short period can reverse stress induced brain damage by stimulating the production of neurohormones. Your body will be able to respond to stress better, which contributes towards feeling happy.

- Brain Boost – Exercise can boost your brain power in several ways to improve memory and build intelligence. Studies show that physical activity on mice and humans will create new brain cells and improve overall brain performance. So, if you have exams to study for, get your HIIT circuits in!

- Increased Confidence – Although the last few paragraphs are here to help you build up your confidence, you will find yourself much more confident once you start making progress towards your goals and start looking good. Be proud of what you have achieved and show off, it's the little things like being able to do 10 burpees without huffing and puffing - while 6 months previously you couldn't even do 5 burpees. This confidence will come naturally, enjoy it!

I think that is enough to persuade you to exercise even if you haven't got a proper goal to work towards. Think of this as a bonus for you reaching your goal, or as your actual goal. With that said, let's move on to more motivation because you can never get enough.

More Motivation

I want for this chapter to a point in which can be read over and over again due to the valuable information included, for this chapter in particular I want for you to re-read this when you haven't got the drive, or you can't be bothered to lay out your fitness mat and complete a HIIT Circuit. This sub-chapter contains a few motivational tips that are different to the ones included in the previous books and will help you get up and get on with it.

Have a Setback Plan – This is where you plan out how to deal with a possible setback like an injury or illness. As unfortunate as a setback is, it should still be planned for because there is always a possibility that you may get injured and you need to know how to deal with the setback. From each injury you pick up you will learn something, once you feel pain you will naturally think back to the potential reasons for the injury - whether it's because you forgot to warm up and you overstretched a muscle during an exercise causing a strain or you were wearing incorrect footwear and slipped on the floor causing a damaged elbow. Once you are injured, you will make a mental note to not do that again, as you know it will cause pain.

A setback plan can contain plenty of information for when you do get injured. Firstly, when you get injured you should be able to focus on what you can and can't do, if it is a serious injury and your doctor tells you to take time off exercise then please listen to them, but if it is a less minor injury then think of ways you can get exercise in without using the injured body part and stick to your previous routine as it can be hard to get back into routine after being out of one for so long – even just walking every day is still exercise. Secondly, focus on your mental health. This is the number one priority because injury can cause stress which isn't needed. Ways in which you can keep a positive mental include surrounding yourself with positive people, doing the things you like (unless it will make your setback worse), getting outside the house and I am sure that you know what helps you best in that situation. Thirdly – don't rush back into training, take your time to let your illness/injury fully go away/heal before training again because if you exercise while unwell or injured it is likely to make matters worse. Finally, you should be able to find rehab exercises which should be gentle and allow for the injured part of your body to be strengthened slowly but surely, so that the rate in which your body can recover from injury increases, meaning that you'll be exercising before you know it.

In the actual setback plan, you should keep a brief note somewhere of what has been suggested previously in a way that is specific to you, so that if you do become injured then you will avoid the negatives that come with the injury - the negatives which may end with further set back and poor mental state – and get back into training as soon as possible. While you are following your setback plan, you should also stick to your healthy diet plan as your body needs the energy to repair, don't let your good habits slip.

Competition – Having a competition amongst friends which is based on reaching fitness goals or any goals is very motivational. As a competitive person myself, I like winning competitions between friends and family even if they are pointless. So, a competition between friends to see who can get their body fat percentage to 5% first, or whatever your goals are, will be very helpful because it will make exercising seem like it has more of a purpose for you and it makes it more fun. This gives you a chance to beat your friends and claim bragging rights!

Routine – A routine is a sequence of actions followed in a sequence. Getting into a training routine is highly motivating because it is something that your body can naturally adjust to. Exercising at certain times in the day, eating 5 times a day with meals 3 hours apart and getting sufficient sleep. Once your body naturally adjusts to your new diet and training plan then it will get easier and feel natural. They say that 3 weeks builds a habit so once you get past the first 3 weeks, you will start completing HIIT Circuits 5 or 6 times a week without thinking about it. If you have to miss a day of training because of unexpected events, then don't stress about it just make sure you don't break your routine for any longer because it is much easier to maintain a routine than break it and have to get back into one.

Learn Positive Self-talk – Think about when a coach or trainer tells you not to give up and keep training, it helps you keep going right? If I was coaching you 1 to 1 then I would be more than happy to support you in this way, but I don't think me writing "C'mon, you can do it!" is as effective as me being there physically to support you. That's why you should learn to encourage yourself, there are many ways in which you can do this – personally I tell myself during a workout "I already know what giving up feels like, so I want to know what it feels like if I don't". Now it doesn't mean you have to say that out loud, that may be a bit awkward in a gym, but think of a way that prevents you giving up, just like how a coach would.

Other motivational tips are in this book and the last two books of this series, some may be more hidden than others, but the idea is that you have much more motivation than you need! Please don't use this motivation to push yourself way too hard, I want you to still stick to your routine as overtraining is linked with a higher chance of injury.

The Comfort Zone

To put this in the best way, you need to push your body to its maximum limit in order to grow towards your goal and see the results. HIIT isn't meant to be easy after all. Although there is something that you should be careful with, and that is pushing yourself way too far out of the comfort zone to the danger zone. As you know, you are likely to be injured if you overtrain but at the same time you need to overtrain to make the gains. That may be very confusing because it's a recipe for injury, but at your fitness level, your body will be able to cope with training at exhaustion for a short period of time – this period of time is where you make the gains. It is only if you try to exercise at exhaustion for a long period of time that you will be at a high risk of injury.

This is something to be careful about, because like mentioned before there is a limit to how far you can get out of your comfort zone. For an example in term of a HIIT Circuit: you could train the HIIT Circuit for an extra 20 seconds, in which you will leaving your comfort zone as you will be at the exhaustion level and this will allow for muscles to be slightly damaged, so that they repair and grow back stronger (causing growth). However, you should not try to train the HIIT Circuit for an extra 2 minutes because your body will be at the point of exhaustion for too long which is very likely to end with a muscle being strained (causing setback). To sum it up nicely, short term discomfort = growth, long term discomfort = danger zone = injury.

I hope that I have helped with this, I am very big on fitness inspiration and I hope to create more in the future to help more people. You may want to read this chapter a couple of times to cement this knowledge in your brain, if you don't agree with any of these tips please let me know in the reviews as I am always looking for ways to improve the quality of my books!

Chapter 9 – Keeping Fit for Life

I have done all I can to help you, it's now your turn to take action with the information that this book provides. Usually at this point, I would say that there is another book that continues from where this is left off, however there is not a next book to this series. There is only so much I can offer, and I don't want to keep repeating myself across these books.

I guess if you have a good prior experience with exercise then you will have a general idea of how you are going to reach your fitness goal. If you are unsure how you are going to reach your goal, then use the six-week training plan from the previous books and use that to get into a routine until you can follow a training plan that satisfies your training requirements. If you are wanting to increase lean muscle mass, don't train circuits that include cardiovascular exercises only as that will only contribute to you losing weight, instead have a mixture of muscular exercises and cardiovascular exercises like squats, push-ups, high knees and so on.

If you are in a position where you cannot complete a HIIT Circuit, then your goal is to complete a HIIT Circuit. Once you reach your goals, that is not a good place to stop, set another one like lowering body fat percentage so you always have something to work towards. The idea is that you should know what you want to achieve, and you should know what will get you there, the hardest part is actually doing it. The previous chapter on motivation should be made easily accessible for you so that if you ever reach a point of struggle you can re-read that chapter for that motivation boost.

As you have made it to the end, I just want to share a secret. This book series was not just a Circuit Training series, the original series was Published last August and contained 4 books. These books were honestly poor, they were around 6,000 words long and each book was completely different, although still under the category of Circuit Training. The books were based on Circuit Training for Beginners (I changed that book and re-published it), Circuit Training - Muscular Strength (Unsavable), Circuit Training – Endurance Training (This one was a load of waffle) and finally Further Circuit Training – HIIT Circuits, which is now this book that has been renamed High Intensity Circuit Training. I managed to turn two books out of that series into this much better series (if I say so myself), the reviews allowed me to make these improvements and that these mistakes are just a part of learning.

So, if you keep making mistakes just like my atrocious book series then just break it down, realise what you are doing wrong and work on improving it – just like I have done with these books. This book series is not perfect by all means, but it is much better and can provide value to readers. Use this as motivation for when things go wrong.

Your Free Gift

The Circuit Training Weight Loss Bundle is a combination of extras to help you reach your goals. These 'extras' can all help in their own way. Below are a few examples of what you may find in this bundle:

- An equipment checklist to help you find all the optional equipment that may help you with HIIT Circuits.

- A calorie tracking app, makes it very easy to split your diet up and keep on track of what you eat.

- An extra HIIT Circuit – this one is what I call the Calisthenics HIIT Circuit.

- A Motivational Poster filled with quotes, something to look at during struggle.

- A HIIT Circuit Cheat Sheet – This makes it easy to refer to the information provided. You may also find a couple other things hidden in the Circuit Training Weight Loss Bundle...

Follow this link to access the free eBook:

https://hudsonandrew.activehosted.com/f/33

Join the Workout for Weight Loss Community

Living a healthy lifestyle is difficult, especially when you feel as if you are doing it all alone. That's why I suggest for you to join a community of others who are in your situation, this community "Workout for Weight Loss" will provide you with daily posts about weight loss and there will be many people that you can talk to, share experiences with and receive help from.

I aim to post twice a day, providing you with tips, tricks, motivation, workouts, diet plans and so much more to help you lose weight. Not to mention that I may host a few book giveaways every now and then. In a community, your chance of reaching your goals is much stronger and you may make many new friends in the process!

So, if you are looking for that extra help, please join my Free Facebook Group: https://www.facebook.com/groups/workoutforweightloss

Conclusion

You have made it to the end of "High Intensity Circuit Training" and I hope this book has either motivated you, has had a positive impact towards your training routine, had a positive effect on your diet, made you learn something new or brought you joy.

This book being the last of the Circuit Training for Weight Loss, I hope that you have all the knowledge to burn fat whether it is to lose weight, lower body fat percentage or exercise for the mental benefits. Below is a brief summary of this book for a brief recap and so it can help you break down the book, so you know which parts to refer to when you need a recap of the information.

This book starts with chapter 1, an introductory chapter to explain what HIIT Circuits are and how they work, which shows the foundations of using circuit training in your fitness routine. Chapter 2 is focused on diet and nutrition and this goes through all the essential nutrients, the structure of a high protein diet, why a high protein diet is most efficient for fat burning, information on the metabolism and the importance of energy. Chapter 3 is all about things that can be done to enhance your training, including training tips, goal setting, injury prevention and progressive overload.

Chapter 4 is more aimed at those who may be experienced with exercise but still want to give HIIT a real good go because HIIT is considered the most effective fat burning training method, this chapter helps those who are not up to the level of HIIT work their way up to completing a HIIT Circuit. Chapter 5 contains the warmups and a cooldown that is used before and after each circuit. Chapter 6 contains the good stuff - the HIIT circuits, there are 5 HIIT Circuits all at different difficulties to provide you with variety.

Chapter 7, this contains the exercise descriptions and a photo for every exercise included in all the circuits. Not only this but there is also a section which explains the benefits of training each muscle to help you understand how the body works and why exercise is important. Chapter 8 is all about motivation where I go into detail about short term discomfort, talk about developing a determined mindset and other positives that exercise can bring to your mental state. Chapter 9, the final chapter which is just a point to suggest how you can use the information in this book to take your training to the next level do you can hit your goals on time.

That's it from me, it's now up to you. Don't forget to check out the Circuit Training Weight Loss Bundle, many benefits in there you can't miss out on!

My Books

The Chump to Champ Collection

Circuit Training for Weight Loss

Reference Page

Dec Beales - Model for the Exercise

Demonstrations.

https://www.instagram.com/dec.beales/

Your Free Gift – The Circuit Training Weight Loss

Bundle.

https://hudsonandrew.activehosted.com/f/33

Join the Facebook Community.

https://www.facebook.com/groups/workoutforw

eightloss

Follow my Facebook Page.

https://www.facebook.com/andrewhudsonbooks

1

Email me for extra support.

andrew@hudsonandrew.com

A.A. (2018a). *Getting a fast metabolism.* Healthline. https://www.healthline.com/nutrition/get-a-fast-metabolism#what-it-is

A.B. (2019a). *Training tips.* Bodybuilding. https://www.bodybuilding.com/fun/10-best-training-tips-ever.htm

A.P. (2017a). *Caffeine before exercise.* Time. https://time.com/4842065/coffee-before-workout-caffeine/#:~:text=Caffeine%20can%20shift%20muscles%20to,its%20efficiency%20in%20generating%20power

Benefits of strong hamstrings. (2017).

Atlaswearables.

https://atlaswearables.com/blogs/atlas/the-

benefits-of-strong-stretchy-

hamstrings#:~:text=Strong%20hamstrings%

20will%20help%20you,various%20ligament

s%2C%20including%20the%20ACL

Coping with injury. (2016). Bodyshotperformance.

https://www.bodyshotperformance.com/how

-to-cope-with-injuries-and-setbacks-in-your-

training/

D.B. (2018b). *Benefits of stretching.* Healthline.

https://www.healthline.com/health/benefits-

of-stretching

D.B. (2018c). *How to measure body fat*. Healthline. https://www.healthline.com/health/how-to-measure-body-fat#:~:text=To%20calculate%20body%20fat%20percentage%2C%20add%20your%20waist%20and%20hip,circumference%20value%20would%20be%2053

Discomfort promotes growth. (2018). Skilledatlife. http://www.skilledatlife.com/why-discomfort-is-good-and-a-sign-of-growth/#:~:text=It%20is%20a%20valuable%20opportunity,she%20can%20achieve%20almost%20anything.&text=The%20discomfort%20we%20feel%20while,are%20getting%20stronger%20and%20healthier

E.K.L. (2017b). *Glucose*. Healthline.

https://www.healthline.com/health/glucose

Foods for better brainpower. (n.d.). Health.Harvard.

Retrieved 2018, from

https://www.health.harvard.edu/mind-and-

mood/foods-linked-to-better-brainpower

Foods for better brainpower. (n.d.). Health.Harvard.

Retrieved 2018, from

https://www.health.harvard.edu/mind-and-

mood/foods-linked-to-better-brainpower

G.M. (2019b). *Benefits of strong triceps*. Healthline.

https://www.healthline.com/health/tricep-

kickbacks#:~:text=The%20triceps%20are%

20essential%20for,and%20increases%20ran
ge%20of%20motion

Good vs Bad carbs. (2017). Everydayhealth.
https://www.everydayhealth.com/diet-
nutrition/diet/good-carbs-bad-
carbs/#:~:text=The%20three%20main%20ty
pes%20of,for%20you%20and%20what's%2
0not

G.T. (2017c). *HIIT benefits.* Healthline.
https://www.healthline.com/nutrition/benefit
s-of-hiit#TOC_TITLE_HDR_3

How to train HIIT. (2018). Inbodyusa.
https://inbodyusa.com/blogs/inbodyblog/ho

w-to-use-hiit-to-improve-your-body-

composition/

J.C. (2019c). *Benefits of strong calves.*

Sportandspinalphysio.

https://sportandspinalphysio.com.au/the-

importance-of-calf-strength-and-the-best-

calf-strength-exercises/

Mental benefits of exercise. (n.d.). Waldenu.

https://www.waldenu.edu/online-bachelors-

programs/bs-in-psychology/resource/five-

mental-benefits-of-exercise

N. (2018d). *Why is a strong back important.*

Integrativeosteopathy.

https://integrativeosteopathy.com.au/build-strong-back-important/

N.B. (2020). *Essential nutrients*. Healthline. https://www.healthline.com/health/food-nutrition/six-essential-nutrients#vitamins

P.R. (2011). *The damage of alcohol*. Bbc. https://www.bbc.com/news/health-15114325#:~:text=Long%20term%2C%20it%20increases%20the,memory%20skills%20and%20reduce%20fertility

Recovery tips. (2018). Clevelandclinic. https://health.clevelandclinic.org/strenuous-workouts-try-these-6-best-recovery-tips/

R.L. (2018e). *Fat burning tips*. Healthline.

https://www.healthline.com/nutrition/best-

ways-to-burn-fat

S.H.Y. (n.d.-b). *Making more time in the day*.

Lifehack.

https://www.lifehack.org/articles/featured/21

-ways-to-add-more-hours-to-the-day.html

S.J. (2016). *Discomfort brings success*. Forbes.

https://www.forbes.com/sites/sujanpatel/201

6/03/09/why-feeling-uncomfortable-is-the-

key-to-success/?sh=5debcaa91913

Using energy. (n.d.). Memorialhermann.

https://memorialhermann.org/services/specia

lties/ironman-sports-medicine-

institute/sports-nutrition/how-the-body-uses-
energy

Why pectoral strength is important. (n.d.).
Trifocusfitnessacademy.
https://trifocusfitnessacademy.co.za/blog/wh
y-pectoral-strength-is-necessary/